HOW TO
SAVE A LIFE:

4/45.

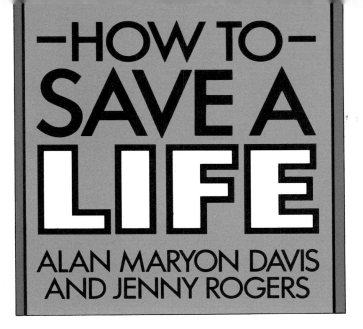

-HOW TO-
SAVE A
LIFE

ALAN MARYON DAVIS
AND JENNY ROGERS

BBC BOOKS

This book accompanies the BBC Television series *Save A Life*, first broadcast on BBC 1 from October 1986. The series was produced by Jenny Rogers and Julian Stenhouse, and presented by Dr Alan Maryon Davis.

Published to accompany a series of programmes prepared in consultation with the BBC Educational Broadcasting Council.

Cover photographs: John Jefford
Illustrations: Will Giles and **(page 104)** Oxford Illustrators

The authors would like to thank Dr David Zideman for his help in preparing this book

Where necessary people's names have been altered to protect their identity

Published by BBC Books,
a division of BBC Enterprises Ltd,
Woodlands, 80 Wood Lane, London W12 0TT

ISBN 0 563 21362 0

This book is set in 11/13 pt Universe
Typeset in England by Redwood Burn Ltd
Trowbridge, Wiltshire
Printed and bound in Great Britain
by Butler and Tanner Ltd, Frome, Somerset

CONTENTS:

❝ *I knew it would happen sooner or later. But I never liked to think about that sort of thing. Somehow I just thought there would always be somebody around who would know what to do.*
Maureen Jones, Leicester, whose husband died of a heart attack, aged fifty three. **❞**

❝ *I just felt awful. Totally useless. If only I'd known then what I know now, I could probably have kept her alive.*
Trevor Hargreaves, lorry driver, Reading, who tried to rescue an eight-year-old girl from drowning. **❞**

❝ *So often, you get to an incident and you find someone dead who could have survived. It especially hurts to see a child or young person who should have had years ahead of them – and what was needed to be done was so simple. Anyone could learn it.*
Dave Fletcher, ambulanceman, Brighton **❞**

6

INTRODUCTION:

There can be few experiences more agonising than being at the scene of a real emergency and not knowing what to do to save a life. It might be a toddler choking; a child drowning; a teenager knocked unconscious; a road accident victim bleeding; or a middle-aged man struck down with a heart attack.

Such emergencies are by no means rare. Every year in Britain about 60 000 people die suddenly and unexpectedly, and it's reckoned that about one in three of such tragedies could be averted if someone on the scene knew the few simple actions needed to keep the casualty alive until medical help arrives.

An emergency can happen anytime, anywhere; and **YOU** might be the person on whom a life depends. What's more, in the great majority of cases, it is likely to be a member of your own family or a close friend whose life hangs in the balance.

WOULD **YOU** KNOW WHAT TO DO?

Many people are reluctant to step in with first aid at the scene of an accident or emergency for fear of making things worse. They may have only the vaguest idea what to do, and perhaps feel that unless resuscitation is performed absolutely perfectly, it's best not attempted at all. But the fact is, when someone's life is at stake and you are the only person around, then it's vital to try to do *something* within a very few minutes.

Time and again, a life is saved by a bystander who, without any formal training, manages to relieve someone's choking, or stem someone's bleeding, or revive someone with mouth-to-mouth breathing. Emergency first aid is largely a matter of common sense and having the gumption to have a go. But obviously it's better to feel confident that what you're doing is helping rather than hindering survival, and that means knowing at least the basics of emergency first aid.

There are now well established simple first aid procedures for all life-threatening emergencies. These have been developed and refined by professionals so that they can be performed by anybody, anywhere, with whatever everyday equipment is to hand. Experts agree that prompt bystander first aid can be as crucial as medical treatment provided by a doctor or ambulance team.

For the first time in this country, a nationwide emergency aid education campaign has been launched – the 'Save A Life' Campaign. This aims to coordinate the teaching of many thousands of people nationwide in the basics of emergency aid through the invaluable work of such organisations as the British Red Cross Society, the St John Ambulance Brigade (St Andrew's in Scotland), the Knights of Malta, the Royal Life Saving Society and others. The Campaign is being spearheaded by the BBC Television series 'Save A Life'.

This book is based on the 'Save A Life' TV series and, like the series, it gives many examples of real life-or-death situations from which people have been rescued by a member of their family, a friend, a workmate or a passer-by. In some cases the rescuer has acted as a direct result of seeing the series and having some idea of what to do. The book gives you not only the practical steps, but also the whys, wherefores and even the feelings you are likely to encounter in a real emergency.

Of course, there is no substitute for going along to a local two-hour class in emergency aid – and there is a 'Save a Life' class somewhere near you (see **p 121** for details). But this book will teach you the principles before you go and will also be a life-long reference aid for you and your family.

Alan Maryon Davis and Jenny Rogers
July 1987

FIRST STEPS IN AN EMERGENCY:

Don't become a casualty yourself

In many emergency situations it can be all too easy to rush to the rescue without making sure that you are not putting yourself, or others, into unnecessary danger. Here are some typical examples:

Road accidents

The main dangers at the scene of a road accident are:
- being run down by approaching vehicles, especially in the dark or fog
- fire, from spilt fuel being ignited by an electrical spark or cigarette
- hazardous chemicals spilt from a tanker

Emergency action at a road accident is dealt with on **p 48**.

Fire

The main dangers to a rescuer are:
- being burnt or overcome by fumes
- becoming trapped in the fire yourself
- being struck by falling timber, masonry, etc.

Emergency action at a fire is covered on **p 95**.

Electrical contact

The main dangers to a rescuer are:
- receiving an electric shock yourself from contact with the casualty
- possible risk of fire

Emergency action for electric shock is dealt with on **p 102**.

Gas and poisonous fumes

The main dangers to a rescuer are:

- risk of explosion and fire in the case of gas
- risk of suffocation or poisoning

Emergency action for gas and poisonous fumes is dealt with on **p 106**.

Drowning

The main dangers to a rescuer are:

- **strong currents**
- **cramp**
- **hypothermia**

Emergency action for drowning is dealt with on **p 77**.

Of course, saving a life may sometimes require an act of heroism. But when there are dangers such as those above, there are usually one or two quick and simple precautions that can eliminate or minimise the risks. It's as well to be aware of these and we have described them in the Emergency Action section of this book **(pp 45–117)**. There is a thin line between heroism and foolhardiness. And two (or more) casualties are a lot worse than one.

Determining priorities

Once you're sure it's safe to approach the casualty, the most important thing is to assess what to do first – see **pp 16–17. Every second counts.**

  If faced with more than one casualty you must assess each one quickly (or as many as you can in about half a minute) before deciding who to tackle first. Assess those who are silent before those who are groaning in response to pain. It is better to achieve as much as you can for as many casualties as possible rather than make a heroic, but all-consuming effort with just one.

CALLING FOR HELP:

Another quick decision you'll have to take is whether you need help and, if so, from whom? Another bystander or passer-by? The casualty's doctor? An ambulance?

It's important to get an **ambulance** in cases of:

- difficulty in breathing
- severe bleeding
- unconsciousness
- suspected heart attack
- serious burns

In the extreme case of heart resuscitation, for example, it has been shown in the USA that it is literally vital to get the ambulance there as soon as possible – preferably within 8–10 minutes. For every minute of delay after that the chances of survival diminish rapidly, despite effective CPR. On the other hand, if the casualty is having difficulty breathing, or is bleeding profusely or is unconscious, he must not be left unattended.

In other words, the cases who need an ambulance most urgently cannot be left while you go for help unless you are confident that their condition is reasonably stable, e.g. the casualty was bleeding heavily but you have managed to control it and he remains conscious; or the casualty is unconscious but you have opened his airway, put him in the Recovery Position and he is breathing well.

The casualty's **GP** may be the best person to call if:

- you've got the GP's name and phone number easily to hand, and . . .
- the problem has happened before and the GP has asked to be called in an emergency, and/or . . .

- you are in a rural area where the GP is much nearer than the ambulance service or hospital.

Usually you will need the help of at least one other bystander to: call for an ambulance (or GP); help you with resuscitation; direct traffic or people clear of the casualty. If necessary, shout at the top of your voice to attract someone's attention, whatever the time of day or night. Don't be afraid of putting people out. **This is an emergency.**

If you do send someone to call an ambulance, make sure they know the important facts:

- exactly where the casualty is
- the casualty's sex, approximate age and, if more than one person is hurt, the number
- the nature of the emergency, e.g. collapsed unconscious, suspected heart attack; fell through glass door, severe bleeding.

Get them to repeat these back to you so that you know they have got the details right. Ask them as well to come back and let you know how long the ambulance will be and help you with the casualty.

Getting an ambulance

The first problem is to find a phone.

If you are in a commercial establishment such as a shop, pub or restaurant, don't be afraid to ask the manager to let you use the phone. This is an emergency and there's no charge for a 999 call. If you're in a public place, such as the street, or a park, it may be quicker to ask at the nearest shop or pub rather than blindly dashing hither and thither looking for a phone box, which may well be out of action if you do manage to find one.

**DIAL 999 AND ASK FOR AN AMBULANCE
REMEMBER – IT'S FREE**

WHAT TO DO:

This is what happens when you dial 999:

1 The emergency operator asks you which service you require.

2 Say 'Ambulance please' even if there is also reason to call the fire brigade or the police. (The emergency operator will call these if necessary.)

3 The operator then rings the ambulance service and will ask you for the number of the phone you are calling from in case you get cut off. This is either on the phone itself or, if you are in a callbox, usually on a notice on the wall, together with the location of the callbox.

4 The ambulance control officer will answer and then ask you for brief details. Be prepared to give the following information and speak slowly and clearly:

- where the incident has happened
- some indication of what has happened (road accident?, bad fall?, drowning?)
- who is hurt or ill (how many?, age?, sex?)
- how badly (severe bleeding?, not breathing?)
- whether there is a fire risk or fumes

5 Once the ambulance is on its way, the control officer may sometimes, if appropriate, give you first aid instructions over the phone. If so, listen carefully.

6 DO NOT PUT THE PHONE DOWN UNTIL THE CONTROL OFFICER HAS DONE SO. HE MAY NEED MORE INFORMATION.

Helping the ambulance find the way

There's little point in the ambulance responding quickly to an emergency call if the driver has to waste precious time finding the way. It's absolutely crucial to give the location of the casualty as accurately as you can. This is relatively easy if it is a building (e.g. someone's home) but can be extremely difficult, for example, on a strange road at night. In the latter case, the phone box you are calling from should have its location written on a notice inside.

While running or driving to the phone, keep an eye out for road signs giving the road number, place names and/or the approximate distance of the casualty to the nearest obvious landmark such as a pub or church.

If possible, you could offer to send someone to the main road or nearby junction or front gate or other appropriate place to look out for the ambulance and direct it.

At night, if indoors, make sure the porch light is on, and you could also open the front curtains and turn the lights on perhaps upstairs and down to make it obvious which house or flat you're in. If possible, flash one set of lights on and off to attract attention.

"

Six-year-old Stephen Saunders and his four-year-old sister Helena found themselves locked indoors when their father knocked himself out in the kitchen. They couldn't open the big bolts on the front or back doors, so Stephen dialled 999.

The ambulance controller asked where they lived but neither of the children knew their full address. Helena knew the road but not the number, so the controller told them to flash the lights in their front room on and off. This signal worked well and the ambulance arrived very quickly. Their father eventually made a full recovery, and the doctors told Mrs Saunders it was entirely thanks to the children that he made it.

"

THE ABC OF RESUSCITATION:

"
John Bunce of Liverpool was a spectator at the Liverpool–Juventus match in Brussels which ended in disaster when part of the crowd pressed against a barrier which collapsed onto another part of the crowd. Many were crushed to death.

John had learned first aid in school swimming lessons and, although injured himself, managed to rescue about a dozen people by dragging them clear and, if unconscious, opening their airway and putting them into the Recovery Position. Nobody else seemed to be helping at all.

He gave one casualty, a girl, mouth-to-mouth breathing until the medical team arrived – she recovered in hospital.
"

ASSESS AND ACT:

Faced with an emergency the key questions are:
- what do you need to do?
- what order do you need to do it in?

In the heat of the moment it's all too easy to waste precious seconds tackling the wrong thing at the wrong time, so here is a checklist of the sequence of vital decisions you will need to make without a moment's delay.

APPROACH
Make sure it is safe to approach the casualty
- see pp 9-10 for potential dangers

CHECK FOR CONSCIOUSNESS
Shake the casualty gently and shout 'Are you all right?' - p 109

NO RESPONSE
Start the ABC sequence of resuscitation opposite

RESPONSE
(even just a groan)
Deal with bleeding - p 58 •
Deal with shock - p 64 •
If semi-conscious,
put in the Recovery Position - p 22, and
keep checking Airway/Breathing/
Circulation • Call for help - p 11

IMPORTANT - Check the consciousness level of *all* casualties before spending time on someone who is conscious.

A for AIRWAY – pp 18-21

Open the casualty's airway - head tilt/chin lift

B for BREATHING – pp 27-34

Look, listen and feel for breathing - p 21

NOT BREATHING

Carry out mouth-to-mouth or
mouth-to-nose breathing - p 28
After 2 breaths, check pulse

BREATHING

Deal with bleeding - p 58 •
Deal with shock - p 64 •
If semi-conscious,
put in the Recovery Position - p 22, and
keep checking Airway/Breathing/
Circulation • Call for help - p 11

C for CIRCULATION – p 35-44

Check to see if the casualty has a pulse - pp 36-37

NO PULSE

Carry out chest compressions - p 37
Maintain rate of 15 compressions
(at 80 a minute), then 2 breaths.
If two people,
5 compressions to 1 breath
Call for help - p 11

PULSE FELT

Continue mouth-to-mouth breathing •
If breathing restarts, place in the
Recovery Position - p 22 •
Keep checking
Airway/Breathing/Circulation •
Call for help - p 11

A FOR
AIRWAY:

The 'airway' is the passage down which air passes to get from the atmosphere into the lungs – in other words, through the mouth or nose to the back of the throat, and then down past the flap of skin at the base of the tongue which shuts over the windpipe when you swallow to stop food going down the wrong way, through the voicebox (Adam's apple) and into the windpipe proper. The windpipe enters the chest and branches into two main air-tubes, one for each lung.

If for any reason a person's airway gets blocked, he will not be able to breathe and will soon suffocate unless the airway is cleared or opened quickly. After a minute or two of obstruction he will start to 'go blue'. After three or four minutes he will start to suffer loss of brain function through lack of oxygen. Shortly after that, his urge to breathe will cease, his heart will stop and he will die.

The airway can become blocked or constricted (narrowed) for several reasons:

- **The tongue may be blocking the throat**

If a person becomes unconscious virtually all the muscles in the body go slack, including the tongue, which can all too easily flop into the back of the throat and block the airway. This is particularly likely to happen if the casualty is facing upwards (whether sitting or lying) because the tongue slips back with the force of gravity. It can also happen as a result of a violent blow in which the tongue gets flung to the back of the throat.

- **There may be pressure on the throat**

If the head falls right forward in a casualty, or an object is pressing on the throat, or the throat is badly bruised or swollen, the airway may be blocked or narrowed.

- **There may be fluid blocking the throat**

In an unconscious person the cough reflex, which makes us cough up anything in our windpipes, does not function, so he may not automatically cough out any fluid or other material lying in the airway. If the casualty is lying face up, any fluid, such as vomit, saliva or blood, will collect in the back of the throat and, if there is enough of it, block the airway.

- **The airway may be blocked by a foreign body**

The casualty may have inhaled something solid such as a lump of food, a piece of broken denture, a bit of a toy, perhaps weeds if he has been under water, which has got stuck in the airway and blocked it (see Choking, **p 84**).

Far too many people die whilst unconscious, completely unnecessarily, just because they are left lying face up, as shown here, with their tongue blocking their airway.

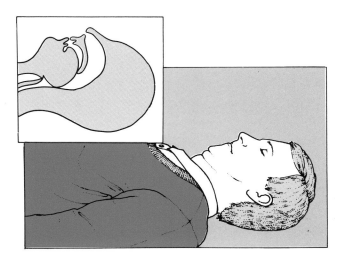

WHAT TO DO:

1   Check to see if the casualty is conscious by shaking him gently and shouting 'Are you all right?'

2   If you get no response, and have no reason to suspect a neck or spine injury (see **p 23**), tilt his head backwards by putting one hand behind his neck to steady it and, with your other hand, *gently* tilting his forehead backwards. This straightens his airway.

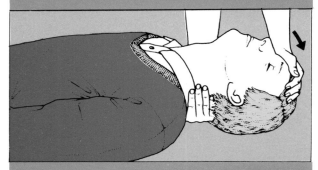

3   Lift his chin upwards by taking your hand from his neck, gripping his chin and lifting it upwards and forwards, leaving the mouth slightly open. This pulls the tongue away from the back of the throat.
This is the open airway position and the casualty should now be able to breathe.

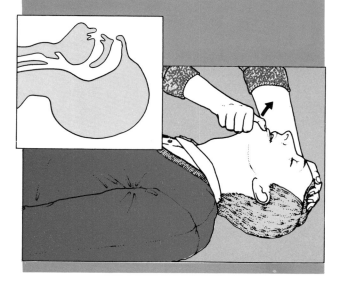

Check – Is the casualty breathing?

Place your ear close to his mouth and nose, and for a few seconds:

LOOK to see if his chest or abdomen is moving

LISTEN for sounds of breathing

FEEL for breath on your cheek

If he is not breathing . . .

Quickly look to see if there is an obvious obstruction in his mouth and, if there is, hook it out with the first two fingers of one hand.

Again, check for breathing
If he is still not breathing . . .
You must start mouth-to-mouth breathing quickly (see **p 28**).

If at any stage the casualty does start breathing . . .
He must be put in a safe position that will keep his airway open and allow any vomit or other fluid to drain out of his mouth, rather than into his lungs. (It is particularly dangerous if acidic stomach juices get into the very sensitive bronchial tubes in the lungs, as these tubes react by producing massive secretions which can clog the lungs completely.)

The simplest safe position is called **The Recovery Position.** If the casualty is unconscious but breathing, put him into the Recovery Position (see **p 22**) and stay with him, checking his breathing, until help arrives. If you need to go looking for help, get back as fast as you can.

THE RECOVERY POSITION:

Perhaps this would be better called *'the life-saving position'* because many emergency experts agree that if there were just one single technique that could be learned about saving lives, this should be it. It is a national tragedy that so many people die quite unnecessarily when they lose consciousness, even for something as comparatively trivial as fainting or concussion, just because no-one around at the time knows how vital it is to put them quickly into the Recovery Position.

An unconscious person lying on her back, or even in a propped-up position, is in very grave danger for three main reasons:

1   Her tongue, like other muscles in her body, will be slack and very likely to slip down the back of the throat, blocking her airway (see **p 18**).

2   Her jaw may be gaping open, putting pressure on the tissues of the throat and constricting the airway.

3   Her protective cough reflex may have failed, and vomit, regurgitated stomach juices, saliva, blood or other fluid may get into the airway and even into her lungs, again narrowing or blocking the airway.

The **Recovery Position** is a safe and stable way of lying so that the airway is kept open and any fluid can drain safely out of the mouth rather than down into the lungs.

> AN UNCONSCIOUS PERSON WHO IS
> BREATHING STEADILY SHOULD BE PUT INTO
> THE RECOVERY POSITION

Exactly how you get someone into the Recovery Position will depend on what position they are in to start with, and also the nature of any injuries they may have. The main worry is whether they have a broken neck or back, in which case you'll need to be extremely careful how you move them so as to minimise the risk of damage to the spinal cord. Otherwise they might end up with further injury.

A broken neck or back is always a possibility if the casualty has:

- been involved in a road accident
- had a bad fall
- had a collision on a sports-field
- hit the bottom of a swimming pool
- suffered any other violent contact

In this sort of situation, it is crucial to avoid over-tilting the head backwards, or bending or twisting the neck or back, whilst trying to get the casualty into the Recovery Position. You've got to keep the head and neck in a straight line and square on as you turn the casualty onto her side. It really takes four people to do this properly, but if there is no help available do the best you can. Once the person is in the Recovery Position, use cushions, pillows or a rolled blanket or rug to keep her there and prevent her from falling onto her stomach.

WHAT TO DO:

Assuming that there is no reason to suspect spinal injury, the casualty is lying on her back and you have knelt alongside and opened her airway to make it easier for her to breathe, you should now:

1 Turn her head gently towards you, keeping it tilted back with the chin forward. If she is wearing glasses, take them off in case they break.

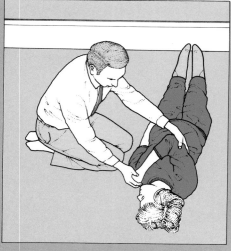

2 Take hold of the arm furthest from you and cross it over her chest. Tuck her hand, palm downwards, under her cheek, ready to act as a cushion.

3 Straighten the arm nearest to you and tuck it, palm uppermost, under her buttock. You'll see why in a moment.

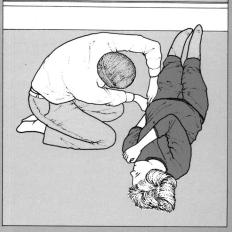

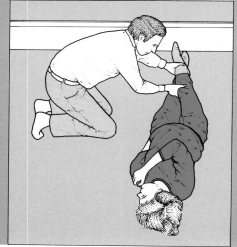

4 Lift the ankle furthest from you and place it across the other ankle.

5 With one hand, grasp her hip, belt or waistband. With the other hand, grasp her shoulder.

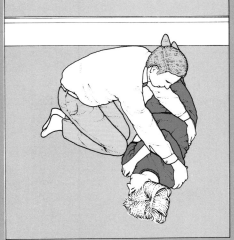

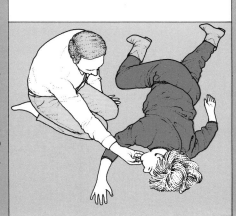

6 Gently roll her towards you onto her side, so that her trunk is resting against your knees, supporting her head as she rolls.

7 Adjust her upper arm to act as a prop for her shoulder and bend her upper leg to prop up her hip. Pull her lower arm out behind her a little to stop her from rolling backwards. Re-adjust her head to keep her airway open.

It's well worth practising this on a friend until you really get the hang of it, and do refresh your memory by re-reading this section from time to time. But in an emergency, don't worry if you can't remember the precise technique – get the casualty into the Recovery Position *somehow*.

Remember – it's best not to leave the casualty alone unless you feel you really must in order to go and find help. And if you do leave her, get back as fast as you can.

❝

Irene Davies probably saved her friend's life when they were in Yugoslavia on a package holiday for the over-60s by taking the right action promptly. This is her story: 'It was a baking hot day – muggy. Margaret and I were in a gift shop browsing around, and we were just looking at some lace when she grabbed my arm and said she felt funny. I just managed to steady her as she buckled at the knees and I let her down gently to the floor. She was out cold on her back.

The shop lady started to flap about and got some cushions to prop her up and I was slapping Margaret's face thinking she must have fainted. But she looked an awful colour and started to make a lot of clicking noises at the back of her throat. That's when it struck me that she couldn't breathe and was probably suffocating on her own tongue. So we took the cushions away and we rolled her onto her side – which took some doing because Margaret's no Twiggy – and straightaway she gave a long gasp and a sort of sigh and started to breathe and her cheeks started to look a better colour.

A minute or two later she came round, completely befuddled and without the faintest idea where she was. But after half an hour she was her old self again and we got a taxi back to the hotel.'

❞

B FOR BREATHING:

You are faced with an unconscious person who does not seem to be breathing.

- You've assessed the situation (see **p 16**).
- You've opened the airway (see **p 18**).
- You've checked for breathing (see **p 21**).

The casualty is definitely not breathing and may be going 'blue' (purple lips and tongue, greyish complexion). Her heart may have stopped. So what do you do?

First, you must use your own breath to get oxygen into the casualty's lungs quickly. This is done by carrying out mouth-to-mouth breathing popularly known as the 'kiss-of-life'; the technical term is *expired air ventilation.*

The air we breathe *in* contains 21% oxygen. The air we breathe *out* still contains about 16% oxygen, which is enough to keep someone alive if we can get enough of it into their lungs, and if their heart is beating properly.

The essence of mouth-to-mouth breathing is to blow regularly, gently and firmly into the casualty's mouth. As you do so, you have to keep an airtight seal on her nose to prevent air from escaping, keep the airway open and make sure that the chest rises and falls with each breath. You also have to check the pulse every now and again. All this sounds rather a tall order, but it's actually a very straightforward sequence and, with proper tuition and practice, you will soon get the hang of it and feel confident.

Although you can practise opening the airway and putting someone into the Recovery Position on a friend, it's best to practise mouth-to-mouth breathing on a training manikin. This is a special plastic dummy that simulates the reactions an unconscious person will usually make to resuscitation. These manikins are available at emergency aid classes (see **p 118**).

WHAT TO DO:

You have to act quickly. An unconscious person who is not breathing will die within a few minutes unless you get enough air into her lungs.

1   Tilt her head back and lift the chin up to open the airway. Look, listen and feel for breathing.

2   If she's not breathing, look quickly to see if there is any blockage in her mouth. If there is, turn her face to one side and, with your first two fingers, quickly sweep it out.

3   Keeping her head back and her chin up with one hand, use the other to pinch her nostrils tight shut. This is to prevent the air you blow into her mouth from escaping through her nose.

4   Take a deep breath, open your mouth wide and seal your lips around her mouth. Blow gently but firmly, without forcing, and at the same time look sideways to watch her chest and see if it rises.

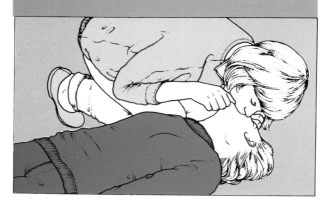

5   Release your mouth and watch the chest fall.

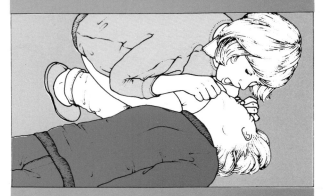

6   *If the chest does not rise:*

- Air may be coming out of her nose. Make sure you keep her nostrils pinched tight.

- You may not be making a tight enough seal with your lips. Open your mouth wider.

- Her airway may not be open enough and the air may be going into her stomach instead. Keep her head tipped well back and her chin lifted up.

- You may not be blowing hard enough or for long enough. Try a firmer fuller breath.

- There may be a blockage further down her airway. Turn her quickly into the Recovery Position and give four firm slaps between her shoulder blades before trying again. Repeat if necessary (see also Choking – **p 84**).

7   If her chest does rise and fall it means the breaths are getting into her lungs, so give **two** full breaths, releasing your mouth between each.

8   If she starts to breathe normally, turn her into the Recovery Position to avoid the risk of her choking on her vomit (see **p 22**).

9   *If normal breathing does not start after your first two breaths:*

- Check her pulse. Her heart may have stopped beating, in which case you must start chest compressions ('heart massage' – see C for Circulation on **p 35**).

10   If you can feel her pulse but she's still not breathing herself, you must keep up the mouth-to-mouth breathing at about 15 breaths a minute until she does breathe again spontaneously, or until medical help arrives. You will know you are winning if her lips and tongue regain their pink colour.

11   If her lips remain blue, double-check your mouth-to-mouth technique, particularly the way you are holding the airway open, and double-check the pulse. If there's any doubt about the latter, start chest compressions.

Young children and babies

You might find a child unconscious and not breathing for many reasons. Some of the most common causes are:

- suffocation, e.g. under pillows, cushions, etc.
- choking on sweets, nuts, bits of toys, pen tops, etc.
- drowning
- some types of severe poisoning
- head injury
- epileptic fit

These are all covered later in this book (see **Index**).

If you are certain or fairly sure of the cause, then you should carry out the appropriate emergency aid for, say, choking (see **p 84**) or a fit (see **p 113**).

But if you really don't know why the child has collapsed and stopped breathing, then you should follow the basic steps outlined above, with a few minor modifications:

- For children under the age of about four, it's best to give mouth-to-mouth-and-nose breathing. In other words, you seal your mouth around the child's mouth *and* nose together.
- Give short gentle breaths.
- Breathe at the rate of about 20 breaths a minute (once every 3 seconds).

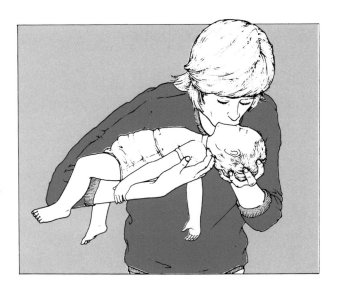

Mouth-to-*nose* breathing

This is an alternative to mouth-to-mouth breathing and has some advantages and some disadvantages.

Advantages

- It may be easier in some situations to seal your mouth around the casualty's nose rather than mouth – for example, if you are in the water with a drowning person.
- You can use both hands to tilt the head back and hold the chin up with the mouth closed, which

31

means you can open the airway to its maximum when blowing in. It's best to open the casualty's mouth to let the air out again.

- You are less likely to over-inflate.
- You are less likely to encounter saliva or vomit.

Disadvantages

- The nose is often too blocked to enable you to get enough air into the chest.
- A nasal injury may make this technique impossible.

Facial injury

A broken nose or jaw, or a severely cut lip or tongue will obviously present difficulties in mouth-to-mouth breathing. Also, if there is facial damage there is an increased likelihood of a broken neck, which means extra special care in any manoeuvring you have to do because of the risk of damaging the spinal cord (see **p 23**).

As far as the injuries themselves are concerned, you must simply do the best you can in the circumstances. It may be messy and very unpleasant, but the victim's life may depend on you making a go of it.

WHAT TO DO:

1   Remove glasses (whether smashed or not) and clear away any broken teeth or dentures.

2   Wipe away as much blood as you can from the mouth and nose area.

3   If possible, hold the edges of a cut lip or cheek together with an improvised swab (e.g. your hanky) or, failing that, your fingers.

"

A seventeen-year-old apprentice engineer, Andrew Forder, was working on some scaffolding, levelling some beams, when he overbalanced and fell, cracking his head on a steel upright, and plunging into a large concrete tank of water, 5 metres deep. He sank like a stone.

While other workmates ran for help, John Redwood, a crane driver, jumped in after him but despite several attempts could not swim down far enough to reach Forder. A few minutes later, Peter Riley, a labourer and a strong swimmer, dived in and at the fourth attempt got Forder to the surface and manoeuvred him out through a channel duct at one end of the tank. He was unconscious, very pale and was apparently drowned.

Another labourer, Philip Allen, who had had some first-aid training, then started mouth-to-mouth breathing and within a minute or two Forder began to breathe unaided. Allen then put him into the Recovery Position where he remained until the ambulance crew arrived.

Despite a fractured skull he made a complete recovery.

"

Concern about AIDS

Many people are concerned that they might catch the AIDS virus when carrying out mouth-to-mouth breathing either on a real casualty or on a training manikin. The only thing we can do is to reassure you that experts have estimated the risk of catching AIDS in either of these ways is less than one chance in a million – in other words negligible. Although it is impossible to be categorical about such a thing, the following facts taken together make it clear that mouth-to-mouth breathing is an extremely safe procedure for the rescuer.

First of all, the AIDS virus is not contagious – this means it does not spread by coughs, sneezes or casual contact such as kissing. Although it has been found in the saliva of people infected with the virus, there has been no known case of anyone catching the AIDS virus from contact with saliva or from a bite-wound. And even in advanced AIDS cases only a very few virus particles can be detected in the saliva. It is simply not present in large enough quantities to pose a threat to a mouth-to-mouth rescuer. Secondly, although the blood of an infected person contains the AIDS virus, there has been no known case of catching AIDS from contact with blood in the mouth.

Finally, despite the widespread anxiety about AIDS it is still an extremely rare condition. Those carrying the AIDS virus are thought to number only about 1 in 1000 of the UK population and virtually all of them are young adults. So, all in all, the risk of catching AIDS from mouth-to-mouth resuscitation of the average casualty is, for all practical purposes, **nil.**

C FOR
CIRCULATION:

If someone's heart stops beating – for example, because they have suffered a massive heart attack – they will immediately collapse unconscious and, after one or two isolated gasps, will stop breathing. Their lips and tongue will go magenta and then purplish through lack of oxygen in the blood. Unless air is got into their lungs and their blood pumped around their circulation within three or four minutes, they will start to suffer irreversible brain damage leading to death.

Alternatively, a person's heart may be beating perfectly well when they first lose consciousness, from drowning, for example, or a heroin overdose, but because they are not breathing, the lack of oxygen in their blood will soon stop their heartbeat. Again, the same emergency resuscitation must be given quickly.

Here is the sort of situation you could find yourself in:

"

When Jane Johnson was walking down Brewery Street at 3.40 pm and came across a man lying in the street, her first reaction was that he was drunk. She looked around her to see if anyone else could help but there was no-one about. The man was purple and his eyes were bulging. She loosened his collar and tie, cleared his mouth and airway, and put him in the Recovery Position (which she remembered from swimming classes several years previously). She then saw that he wasn't breathing, so she started mouth-to-mouth and heart massage. Two people walked past and ignored her request to telephone an ambulance. Jane carried on, thinking 'Why me? Why me?'

Eventually a youth arrived who seemed to know what to do and took over the chest compressions. Together they worked on the man for another 20 minutes and his colour started to improve. The police arrived and said they were doing well and called an ambulance.

Jane was convinced the man was dead when they took him away, but later the police phoned her to say that he was recovering in the coronary care unit.

"

You are faced with someone who is lying unconscious — let's say it's a middle-aged man. You quickly assess the situation (**p 16**), open his airway (**p 18**) and look/listen/feel that he is not breathing (**p 21**). You give the two initial mouth-to-mouth breaths (**p 29**). This has no effect; his pupils are widely dilated and he looks dead.

NOW WHAT DO YOU DO?

You must check his pulse

You have to find out quickly if his heart has stopped beating. It's no good feeling for a pulse at the wrist because he is likely to be in a state of shock (i.e. his blood pressure has dropped dramatically) and so the circulation to his limbs will be restricted. Even if his heart is still beating you probably won't be able to feel it at the wrist.

The place to feel for a pulse is in the neck. The two main arteries to the brain, the carotid arteries, lie in the grooves on either side of the voicebox or Adam's apple. These arteries are about the last to shut down when the circulation fails.

How to feel for the pulse

With your middle two fingers, press deep into the groove on one side of the windpipe under the chin. You should be able to feel a strong regular pulse. (Try it on yourself now.) Because it may be weak or irregular in an unconscious person, it's important to allow several seconds before assuming it has stopped.

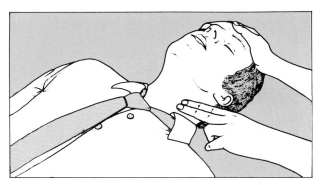

Finding a casualty's pulse.

IF YOU CAN'T FEEL A PULSE, YOU **MUST** START
CHEST COMPRESSIONS IMMEDIATELY

Chest compression

Colloquially known as 'heart massage', but properly called *external chest compression*, this is a simple and effective way of keeping a casualty's blood circulating when his heart has stopped beating. Of course, chest compressions are nothing like as effective as real heartbeats, pumping round only a third of the normal amount of blood. Nevertheless, providing air is being put into the lungs (e.g. by mouth-to-mouth breathing), chest compressions can be enough to keep the body supplied with enough oxygen to keep going and for the casualty to recover.

What chest compressions actually do is to use the natural springiness of the rib-cage to squeeze the heart

between the breastbone and the backbone and then release it. Because the heart has one-way valves, the blood
it contains gets forced out into the main arteries with each
compression, and blood rushes in from the main veins
with each release. In other words, with each compression
and release, blood circulates a little. And if the compressions are kept up at the rate of about 80 a minute, with two
mouth-to-mouth breaths after every 15 compressions, a
reasonably satisfactory blood pressure can be maintained
(about two thirds of the normal level), circulating reasonably well oxygenated blood.

The technique

The technique of chest compression is actually quite
simple, once learned. But it is important to get it precisely
right for it to be really effective and not cause unnecessary injury. Having said that, if someone's heart has
stopped beating, any attempt at chest compression is
better than none at all.

Ideally the casualty should be lying flat on his back on a
firm surface, e.g. the floor or ground. If he's on a springy
mattress, however, and it's difficult to move him, try to
pull him to the edge of the bed where the mattress should
be harder.

The compression has to be applied to the correct spot
on his chest, **i.e. on the middle of the lower half of his
breastbone.** There are two easy ways to find this:

1 Feel for the notch at the top of his breastbone (between the ends of the two collar-bones) and also the
notch at the lower end of his breastbone (where the
bottom ribs meet in the middle) and find the halfway point
between these two notches. Then find the *middle of the
lower half* of the breastbone. That's the spot to place the
heel of your hand (see opposite).

2 Alternatively find the notch at the lower end of the
breastbone, measure two fingers' width up from there
(3–4cm, 1–1½ inches) and place the heel of your hand at
that point on the breastbone (see opposite).

The reason for all this precision is that, firstly, that is the point of maximum leverage or 'travel' on the breastbone and is also directly over the heart, and secondly, heavy pressure to either side of that spot could easily break a rib, or below that spot could rupture an abdominal organ.

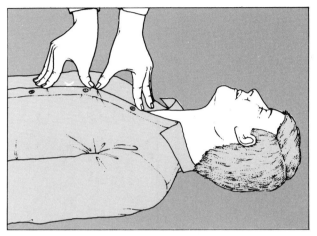

Method 1: Finding the middle of the lower half of the breastbone. X marks the spot for compression.

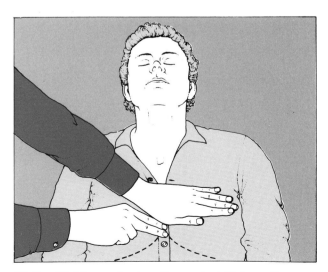

Method 2: Measuring two fingers' width from the lower notch.

WHAT TO DO:

1 Make sure you are positioned comfortably kneeling beside the casualty, level with the compression spot. Put the heel of one hand on it, and the heel of your other hand on top of that, interlocking your fingers but holding them off the chest (see below).

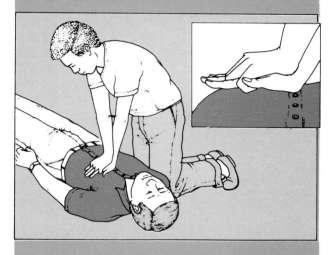

2 Lean forwards, with your head and shoulders directly above the casualty's chest. *Keeping your elbows straight,* push firmly and steadily down on the breastbone, compressing the chest by about 4–5cm (1½–2 inches) and immediately releasing.

3 Repeat this to a count of 15 at a rate slightly faster than one a second (80 per minute). It helps to say out loud, 'One-and-two-and-three-and-four-and-etc' up to 15.

4 Then move to the casualty's head and give two full breaths using mouth-to-mouth breathing (see **p 28**).

5 Then back to the chest again for another 15 compressions followed by two breaths.

6   Check the pulse after the first minute of compressions and mouth-to-mouth (i.e. four cycles), and every three minutes after that.

7   Keep up this rhythm until help arrives; or the casualty's heart starts beating again. It's certainly hard work but it's vital that you keep going. People have made full recoveries even after hours of CPR (*cardiopulmonary resuscitation*, i.e. mouth-to-mouth breathing and chest compression).

If you start to feel a pulse

Stop chest compression but carry on with the mouth-to-mouth until the casualty starts breathing on his own again.

When this happens, turn the casualty into the Recovery Position (see **p 22**) and keep checking pulse and breathing until help arrives.

A few dos and don'ts

● **Do** feel for the pulse in the neck rather than the wrist.

● **Do** be as sure as you can that the heart has stopped beating before you start chest compressions. Chest compressions on a beating heart can sometimes upset its rhythm, making matters worse. On the other hand, without a heart monitor machine (ECG) you can never be absolutely certain, and if the casualty's colour (lips and tongue) stay purple despite mouth-to-mouth breathing, and his pupils are widely dilated, then you must assume the worst and get pressing.

● **Do** position your hands correctly on the breast bone.

● **Do** lock your fingers together and keep them off the chest. Only the heel of your lower hand should actually be touching the chest. This avoids spreading the pressure, which could break ribs.

● **Do** keep your arms straight and your shoulders directly above the chest.

- **Don't** bounce or jerk. Pressure should be a steady downward thrust and release, and you should only be moving at your hips and knees.

- **Don't** overdo it: 4–5cm (1½–2 inches) movement is all that's needed. More could cause damage.

- **Don't** forget to count, '*One, and, two, and, three, and four, etc.*' to fifteen, then give two breaths, and repeat.

- **Don't** forget to check the pulse after the first minute and then every three minutes after that.

- **Do** get some practice at all this. By all means try it on cushions or a pillow, but there's no substitute for the special training manikins available at classes and the personalised tuition that goes with them (see **p 118**).

- **Don't** practise on a living person.

BUT above all

- **Don't** feel that it's all too complicated and you'll never get the hang of all these do's and don'ts. It's actually much more straightforward than it sounds. And if faced with an emergency . . .

DO HAVE A GO

If someone else is with you

If there is someone else around and you know the ambulance is on its way, get them to help you. One of you should do the mouth-to-mouth breathing and pulse-checking whilst the other does the chest compressions. Swap round every now and again; pressing a chest is very tiring. Keep a steady rate of compressions at one a second, but with a momentary pause on the upstroke of every *fifth* compression for the helper to give *one* breath. This is considered to be the best routine possible for getting oxygen into the blood and circulating it; the different routine when you are working alone is a necessary compromise.

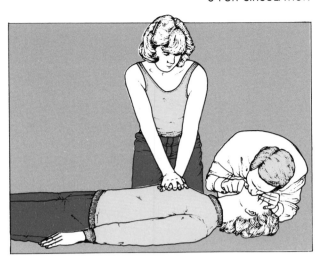

When there is someone to help you, give 5 compressions for each breath. Swap tasks every few minutes.

66

Two hanggliders collided with each other 100 feet above the Sussex Downs and crash-landed on a grassy hillside near a group of spectators. One of the spectators, a trained first-aider, ran down to the pilots and found one of them to be deeply unconscious, not breathing and without a pulse. The spectator immediately started CPR and was joined by another spectator who helped with the mouth-to-mouth breathing.

After less than a minute the pilot's pulse returned and he began to breathe on his own. They put him in the Recovery Position and by the time an ambulance had arrived, about 20 minutes later, the pilot was conscious enough to ask what had happened. His only physical injury was a broken jaw.

99

Babies and small children

Although the same principles apply when resuscitating a baby or small child, you have to use a slightly different technique with faster but much less forceful movements.

● Give mouth-to-mouth-*and-nose* breathing using *gentle* puffs at a rate of about *20 per minute,* checking for the pulse after *two* breaths.

● Do chest compressions using *two fingers* pressing on the *lower half* of the breastbone (one finger's breadth up from the bottom notch), at a rate of *at least 100 per minute,* pushing it down about 1–2.5 cm (½–1 inch). The ratio is *5 compressions to 1 breath.*

Older children

Again, faster and gentler movements are the rule.

● Mouth-to-mouth-*and-nose* breathing is best for younger children, standard mouth-to-mouth for older ones, at *20 breaths per minute,* checking for the pulse after *two* breaths.

● Chest compressions should be done with *one hand only*, at a rate of about *100 per minute*, pushing down on the lower half of the breastbone to a depth of 2.5–4cm (1–1½ inches). The ratio for children over 6 is *15 compressions to 2 breaths.*

EMERGENCY ACTION:

"

Maurice Garden of Nottingham was cycling home one evening when he heard a bang and saw a car screeching to a halt in front of him with a white object stuck under the front of it. He dismounted, ran to the car and carefully pulled out the 'object', a three-year-old boy, Justin Wolfe. The car driver ran to get help.

Justin was unconscious and had a serious head wound which was bleeding profusely. Mr Garden applied direct pressure to the wound with his handkerchief and managed to stem the flow, but then noticed that Justin was not breathing and had gone blue. Mr Garden had read about resuscitation in a magazine and started mouth-to-mouth breathing. After a few minutes Justin began to breathe of his own accord again and his colour returned. An ambulance arrived and took him, still unconscious, to hospital where he subsequently recovered.

"

ROAD TRAFFIC ACCIDENTS:

A road traffic accident can indeed be a terrifying, messy emergency and one calling for all the resources of knowledge, calm and leadership that you possess. By tradition, this is the scene that shrieks 'leave it to the professionals', precisely because it looks so frightening. The following is one young woman's experience of just such a scene:

> **"**
>
> I was driving home from a party late one winter night and I passed an accident just off the motorway. I did at least stop and get out. The two cars were both wrecked. There was glass all over the road. A little girl was being sick on the verge. Two young men who were passengers were wandering about – one of them was crying. There was a lot of blood everywhere. The front passenger in one of the cars was trapped inside and looked terrible, but I didn't know what to do – I felt sure that she shouldn't be moved because you always hear such a lot about the danger of spinal injuries. Other motorists had stopped, so I found out that the ambulance, etc., were on their way. I was thankful to get in my car and drive off. Afterwards I felt pretty awful about my feebleness . . . in fact it was my main reason for doing a first aid course later. Now I realise how stupid it was not to ask if I could do anything, but ignorance made me terrified of making things worse.
>
> **"**

Even if this young woman had attempted to make a more positive contribution at this accident, there might have been no need to do more. Perhaps the trapped casualty was conscious; perhaps the other bystanders had already done everything that could be done before the emergency services arrived. Fear of 'making things worse', however, prevented her, like many others, from assessing the scene herself. A simple intervention such as turning off the crashed cars' ignition, or supporting the casualty's airway, might have been life-saving.

Here is a completely different reaction to an equally frightening scene. David Morgan, an architect in Leicester, was one of the first people to take a 'Save A Life' class at the beginning of the campaign. Only a few days after doing the class, he was able to come to the aid of a woman pedestrian knocked unconscious by a car on a wet winter evening:

"

She was lying huddled in the road half on her side and her head was collapsed towards her chest. She was covered in blood and there were several other people standing around looking helpless. I bent over her as I'd been taught to do and gently shook her – it was obvious she was unconscious and I listened and looked for breathing and couldn't hear or see any, but I found her pulse which was slow. I gently rolled her over to open her airway, and as I did so she gave a 'hurrumph' sort of noise – a bit like a horse. She gave a great gasp after that and started breathing on her own. I'm quite sure that only a week before I'd have felt that I mustn't touch her. As it was, I knew that, since she was unconscious, it was important to get her tongue off the back of her throat. I just did it all automatically – I didn't stop to ask myself whether I should or shouldn't intervene.

"

Mr Morgan's actions were life-saving; this casualty would almost certainly have died without his help – not from her injuries which turned out to be fairly minor, but from suffocating on her tongue because she was unconscious.

The priorities

Unlike many other kinds of emergency first aid, a road traffic accident is complicated by the fact that the setting itself is potentially dangerous to the rescuer. Many accidents happen on exceptionally busy roads, at night and in conditions where bad weather makes it difficult for other drivers to anticipate trouble.

WHAT TO DO:

1 **Be safe yourself.** Park your car behind the crashed cars and switch on your hazard lights. This gives other motorists some warning of danger. Set up a warning triangle if you have one. Ask another bystander to help direct traffic around the accident. If you are wearing a dark coat and something light underneath, take the coat off: that way you will be seen more easily.

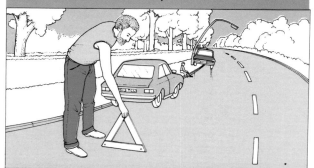

2 **Prevent fire.** Turn off the ignition in crashed cars. Check that handbrakes are on. Diesel lorries and buses often have a clearly labelled emergency fuel supply switch outside the vehicle. Switch it off. Don't let anyone smoke.

Many vans and lorries carry dangerous chemicals. These vehicles must display special 'Hazchem' panels. If they are likely to catch fire spontaneously, the panel includes a flame symbol. It will also give a code number and a telephone number.

Only approach a vehicle carrying a Hazchem panel with the greatest caution and *only* if the driver urgently needs help. Dial 999 and pass on all the details.

3   **Assess the casualties.** Appearances can be deceptive. A casualty who is shouting or crying is usually less seriously injured than one who is merely moaning. The totally silent casualty is the one most likely to need your attention, as her breathing and pulse may have stopped.

Look carefully all over the car: there may be a baby who has rolled out of a carry cot and underneath a seat. You should look outside the car too. In some accidents, people are thrown over hedges. One young motorcyclist was recently the victim of such an accident, but survived for several days, keeping himself alive by sucking grass for moisture before he was finally discovered.

If there are conscious casualties, ask them how many people were in the car.

4   **Help the most seriously injured first.** This is the best order of priority for treating victims: Unconscious, not breathing: apply CPR (**pp 18–43**). Bleeding severely: control it (**p 60**). Unconscious but breathing: turn into the Recovery Position (see **p 22**). Conscious but shocked: treat for shock (**p 64**).

5   **Don't move a trapped casualty** unless you absolutely must because of danger from fire or because breathing and heartbeat have

stopped. The risk of neck or spinal injuries is high in road and traffic accidents. Ambulance personnel are trained in the special techniques needed to move such casualties.

6 Send for help. Send another bystander to dial 999 (**p 12**) while you are giving first aid. Motorways have free telephones every mile. Encourage this helper to flag down another car if necessary to save time. Don't worry about whether someone else has already called the emergency services: it is better to make certain that someone is dialling 999 than to risk the possibility that no one has. Never cross a motorway to an emergency telephone: the chances of being both cause and victim of a fresh accident are far too high.

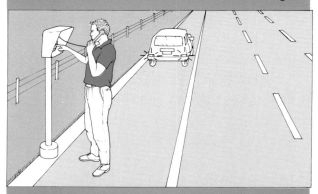

7 Help the emergency services. Tell ambulance personnel what you have observed and what help you have given. The police will want to know if you witnessed the accident. If your own vehicle has been directly involved, you need to:

- Exchange names and addresses with the other driver.
- Note his or her car registration number.
- Exchange car insurance details.
- Note names and addresses of witnesses.

50

What if I have to take charge?

The question underlying this question is, '... and if I do, will anyone take any notice?' In reality, this difficulty is unlikely to arise:

> **"**
>
> *I am a pretty mousy person most of the time: I hate being conspicuous. It really surprised me that when I had to take control of a nasty accident because no one else seemed to know what to do, everyone just did as I asked. One of the people just standing around gawping was an officious-looking middle-aged man who kept saying over and over again, 'Someone should do something.' I calmly told him to go off and call 999 and he just meekly did it. I was amazed that so many people were saying, 'Don't touch them, don't touch them.' I felt that I knew what to do and I found it came quite naturally to give other people instructions.*
>
> **"**

Other people find that, even if they are quaking inside, a calm exterior or the appearance of authority is enough to instil confidence in others:

> **"**
>
> *I'd always assumed that you would need a uniform or a little black doctor's bag to take charge, but this isn't so. I arrived to find about six other people dithering and panicking. They were only too pleased to have someone there who knew a bit of first aid, even though I must have been the youngest there by fifteen years. I was very frightened inside, but I knew that I was putting on a pretty convincing act on the outside.*
>
> **"**

What if the victim is trapped?

We have already explained that you should not attempt to move a trapped casualty in a road accident because of the danger of spinal or neck injury. The casualty may also have a broken limb: moving it unthinkingly may cause serious internal bleeding.

However, this does not mean you should do nothing. An unconscious casualty will die unless you maintain his airway. You can do this without dragging the casualty out of the car. Open the airway and support the chin until skilled help arrives.

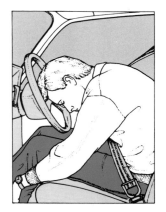 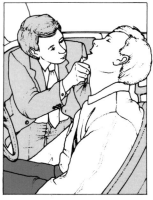

Even if you can't move a car accident victim, you can still open his airway and ensure he is breathing.

Learning this simple technique meant that Phil Genlloud knew what to do when she came across an accident on a country road in Lincolnshire:

❝

There were two cars slewed across the road. The driver of one was already being helped by someone who had arrived before me. This man said, 'This one's all right, but I don't think we can do anything about the other chap, he looks a goner to me.' I went round to

*the driver's side of the other car which was
making a horrible noise, hissing and spitting
and clicking. The engine was still running, so
I switched it off. The driver was slumped so
that his head was jammed against the steer-
ing wheel. His face was blue and he didn't
seem to be breathing. I'd done first aid on a
mountain rescue course years before, and I
remembered about opening the airway. So I
just gently lifted his head and supported his
jaw. As I did it, he gave a snort and gasp, and
I heard air rushing in. I kept supporting his
chin and after a bit he began moaning and
coming round. He was nearly conscious by
the time the ambulance arrived.*
99

A *conscious* casualty can be comforted and reassured
until the emergency services arrive. Don't give him anything to drink: an anaesthetic may be needed later and a
drink may cause vomiting.

What if the victim's breathing and pulse stop?

If there is no sign of breathing or pulse when you have
ensured that the airway is clear, you have no choice but to
move the casualty. He will die unless you give CPR, and to
give CPR you must move him. Putting it crudely, your first
priority must be to save life: better a live patient with a
possible spinal injury than a dead one.

What if I must move the casualty?

If you must move a casualty because of fire danger or
because breathing and pulse have stopped, this is the
method to use. You must have a helper whose role is to
steady the head, keeping it in a straight line with the body.

WHAT TO DO:

1 Work from the nearest open car door. Bend the victim's arm across her chest, then squat just behind her, slide your arms through her armpits and grasp her bent forearm with both your hands.

2 Get your helper to hold the casualty's head, keeping it in line with her body as you move.

3 You and your helper should then move slowly and steadily backwards, carrying the casualty clear of the car.

What if I'm on my own?

The basic rule of all emergency first aid is to give help first, then to dial 999 when you are sure it is safe to leave a casualty unattended. The reason is that if a victim is unconscious and not breathing, the time taken to call an ambulance takes away time from the vital few minutes when resuscitation is possible. In reality, a road accident is always a public event. Shortage of possible helpers is not usually the problem, and most bystanders, or uninjured passengers, will be glad of something positive to do.

What if it's a motor-cyclist and he's wearing a helmet?

Motorcyclists are the most vulnerable of all road users. The fact that they are mostly inexperienced young men who enjoy taking risks is compounded by the lack of protection afforded by their bikes. The basic rule about helmets is leave them on if you can because of the danger of neck injury. Remove them only if the casualty is:

- Not breathing.
- Vomiting.

In these cases you must get the helmet off to save his life.

Head-only helmets

Cut through or release the chinstrap. Force the sides of the helmet apart and lift the helmet upwards and backwards.

Full-face helmets

1 Ask a helper to support the casualty's head and neck while you are removing the helmet.

2 Tilt the helmet up and back until it is clear of the chin.

3 Now tilt the helmet **forwards** until the upper part comes over the forehead.

4 Lift the helmet off.

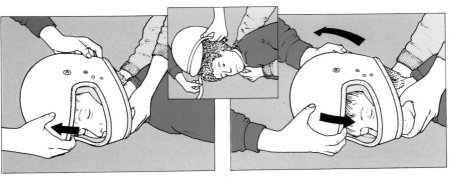

Removing a full-face helmet.
Inset: Removing a head-only helmet.

The reality

Most road traffic accidents are messy and frightening. They often involve more than one casualty; there is likely to be a lot of crumpled metal, broken glass, blood and crying. The reality of giving first aid is nothing like the clean, controlled atmosphere of a first aid class. Be prepared for it to be both distasteful and upsetting. The man whose experience is quoted below won an award from the Royal Humane Society for his prompt help in an emergency, but he found that the whole episode haunted his thoughts for many months afterwards, not least perhaps because it was not the neat 'heroic' event that might have been imagined.

"

I was at home when I heard a tremendous bang outside. I looked out of the window and saw that a child had been knocked down by a car which was now wrapped round a lamp post. One of my neighbours was putting a cushion under his head and I thought, 'I can do better than that – he's blocking the airway.' I went outside. The boy was blue and wasn't breathing. He didn't have a pulse so I started giving CPR. I went on for about fifteen minutes, though it seemed like an hour, and I discovered later that one of the other bystanders was a nurse. What surprised me was that the boy felt so small and fragile. I had practised on a manikin at my first aid class, but this felt quite different. After about fifteen minutes I noticed some signs of life. Then suddenly the boy vomited into my mouth. I looked up and saw someone standing there. He was wearing white and I thought he was an ambulanceman, though actually it turned out that he was a fireman. I told him to put the boy into the Recovery Position. I went back into my house and vomited copiously myself. The papers and police gave this fireman all the credit for saving this boy's life, which I didn't think was right. The boy sustained a bad head wound and had some brain damage, but he actually made a fair recovery, so I think it was all worth it.

"

Equipped for trouble

A first aid kit in itself does not guarantee that you will be able to give appropriate help. *Knowledge* of emergency first aid procedures is always going to be more useful than a few bandages. However, it is reassuring to know that you can carry some general rescue equipment in your own car. The most useful items are:

● **Torch:** for signalling to other cars; to search for casualties, check car ignition, etc.

● **Blanket:** to cover shocked casualties. Emergency foil 'blankets' are useful, cheap, and can be folded into a small packet.

● **Hazard triangle:** to act as advance warning of a car breakdown or accident.

● **Fire extinguisher:** make sure that this is suitable for fires in cars.

● **First aid box:** a plastic, airtight kitchen box is ideal. Fill it with a selection of bandages, sterile dressings, cotton wool, adhesive strip, a pair of scissors and a few safety pins.

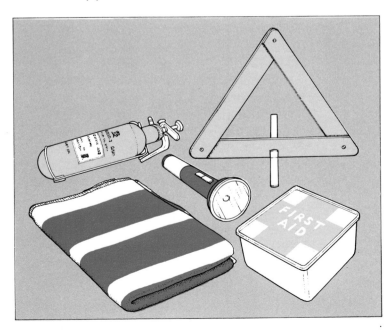

BLEEDING:

Massive bleeding (technically referred to as *haemor-rhage*) is not only a serious threat to a casualty's life, it can also be extremely frightening for you as the potential life-saver. Many people feel faint at the sight of blood, especially bright red blood, spurting out of a wound in large quantities. For some, just the thought of it is alarming.

However, it is just that sort of injury which is most life-threatening and which requires a quick and purposeful reaction – despite the panic and the mess. If the bleeding is that fast, there's no time to run for help. You have got to stop it, or at least slow it down, before the casualty bleeds to death.

This eyewitness account describes how prompt action stopped a casualty's heavy bleeding:

"

As the train came to a standstill, a girl in her teens ran along the platform and was struck hard by a door swinging open. She clutched her forehead and bright blood gushed out between her fingers. She staggered and knelt down as commuters rushed past her. One side of her face and hair was just a mass of blood, which seemed to be squirting from her eye. After what seemed ages, but was probably just a minute or two, a middle-aged lady rushed up and pressed her hanky on the girl's temple and made her lie down. That seemed to stop the bleeding. It turned out she'd severed an artery in her temple, but her eye was all right.

"

The average adult man has about 5 litres (8 pints) of blood circulating in his body, a woman a little less, and children a lot less, depending on their size. The volume of blood is kept under constant control by special sensors in the circulatory system. If a relatively small amount of blood is lost – say, by donating a pint to the transfusion service – the body reacts by diverting fluid from the tissues into the bloodstream to make up the lost volume, which takes a few hours. And over the next few days the bone marrow makes extra blood cells to replace those lost.

However, if a lot of blood is lost suddenly, this process is far too slow. As the amount of blood in the system lessens, the blood pressure drops and the casualty becomes pale, sweaty and feels giddy and faint. This is called 'shock' (nothing to do with electricity). In a case of severe shock the blood pressure may drop so low that not enough blood reaches the brain and the casualty passes out. If unconsciousness deepens further, breathing and heartbeat will soon stop and death will be inevitable, unless blood or plasma can be given very quickly, together with cardiopulmonary resuscitation (CPR – see **p 37**).

There are three main types of bleeding, depending on the type of blood vessels damaged.

Arterial bleeding

Blood in the arteries is under pressure and therefore spurts out in time with the pulse. Arterial blood looks bright red, and if a main artery is severed (for example, the *femoral* artery in the groin), a lot of blood can be lost very quickly indeed. Smaller arteries (such as those in the hand) have the ability to constrict (narrow) and so help to reduce blood loss.

Venous bleeding

Blood in the veins is under low pressure and pours steadily out of a wound. Nevertheless, if a large vein is cut or torn (for instance, a varicose vein), again a lot of blood can be lost. Venous blood is dark red.

Capillary bleeding

Blood in the capillaries (microscopic blood vessels) is at virtually zero pressure and simply oozes or drips slowly from superficial cuts and grazes. This flow usually ceases after a few minutes as the capillaries clamp shut and the blood clots, forming a seal.

Controlling blood loss

The faster the flow of blood from a wound, the greater the risk of shock to the casualty, and also the less likely it is that a clot will be able to form quickly enough to plug the leak before it gets washed away.

The aims of emergency aid are therefore to stop blood loss and to stem the flow long enough for clots to form in the damaged vessels. There are two main ways of helping to achieve this:

Applying pressure. This usually takes the form of direct pressure on the wound. It has to be firm enough to compress the blood vessel(s) concerned in order to stop or restrict blood flow. (Much more pressure is needed for an artery than for a vein.) It also has to be kept up long enough for vessel constriction and clotting to take place (usually 10 to 15 minutes).

In rare cases it may be necessary to apply *indirect* pressure – that is, at a point other than the wound itself. For instance, in the case of a limb which is seriously wounded in a number of places, with very bad arterial bleeding, it may be best to press down hard over the main artery for that limb at a point where it lies against a bone. In the arm this should be done where the main artery passes down the inner surface of the upper arm bone; in the leg where the main artery passes over the front rim of the pelvis in the middle of the groin crease. Because such pressure on the main artery acts like a tourniquet, shutting off the blood supply to the whole limb, it should only be used in dire circumstances and *should not be maintained for longer than 15 minutes.*

Raising the wound above the level of the heart. This helps to reduce blood loss from veins and capillaries by reducing the pressure in them.

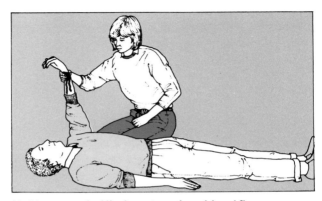

Hold a wounded limb up to reduce blood flow.

WHAT TO DO:

1 Simply press firmly on the wound with your fingers, holding the edges together. If the cut or tear is large, you may need to use both hands to hold the edges together and maintain pressure.

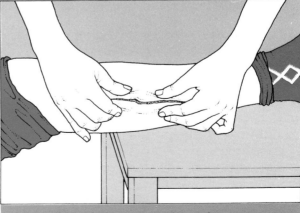

Hold the sides of a large wound together.

2   Lay the casualty down if you can and raise the injured part as far as you can above the heart.

3   After 10 to 15 minutes, carefully release pressure to see if bleeding has stopped, or nearly stopped. If it has, make a pad of sterile gauze, larger than the wound, and bind it in place with a firm (but not over-tight) bandage. If no gauze is available, you can use a clean handkerchief, paper tissues or similar material. For a bandage you can use a scarf, pair of tights or necktie. If the pad becomes soaked with blood, *don't remove it,* because that might disturb the clot. Instead, place another pad on top of the original and bandage it firmly in place.

4   If blood loss is enough to cause shock, treat this as outlined in the next section.

Internal bleeding

Internal bleeding can be caused by a heavy fall, road accident, deep-penetrating wound, crush injury, or medical condition such as a perforated peptic ulcer. Whenever a bone is broken or an organ ruptured, internal bleeding is a possibility.

Although the bleeding is within the body, blood is still being rapidly lost from the circulation. Indeed, internal bleeding is often more life-threatening than external bleeding because it is harder to detect and more difficult to control.

The most obvious symptoms and signs of sudden severe internal bleeding are those which accompany shock (see **p 64**).

Other problems are caused when bleeding into a confined space within the body puts pressure on vital organs, particularly if the bleeding is from an artery. Bleeding inside the skull, for example, can put enough pressure on the brainstem (the connection between the spinal cord and the brain) to be fatal. Bleeding into the chest cavity can put severe pressure on a lung, causing breathlessness.

Sometimes internal bleeding is revealed by blood appearing at the surface: for instance, bleeding from the nose or ear in the case of a fractured skull; vomiting 'coffee grounds' blood from a bleeding peptic ulcer; passing bright red blood with the stools from bleeding piles (*haemorrhoids*); major bleeding from the vagina of a pregnant woman due to a ruptured placenta. In some cases of bleeding within the chest or abdomen, widespread mottled bruising of the skin can occur.

As with external bleeding, if more than about a quarter of the total blood volume is lost, the casualty can become severely shocked.

WHAT TO DO

1 Treat for shock if necessary (see **p 64**).

2 Get someone to call for an ambulance.

3 Keep a check on the casualty's level of consciousness, breathing and pulse.

4. If the casualty passes out but keeps breathing, put him into the Recovery Position (see **p 22**).

5 If the casualty stops breathing, carry out mouth-to-mouth resuscitation (see **p 28**) and keep a check on his pulse.

6 If his heart stops, carry out chest compressions (see **p 37**) and mouth-to-mouth breathing until medical help arrives.

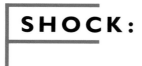

SHOCK:

Shock is an emergency condition in which the normal flow of blood throughout the body suddenly becomes reduced, so that the brain and other vital organs are deprived of oxygen, leading to giddiness or loss of consciousness. There are three basic causes:

1   The heart may suddenly lose its pumping power.
This can happen, for example, after a severe heart attack.

2   The amount of blood in the circulatory system may be suddenly reduced. This can result either from loss of blood itself, or indirectly through severe loss of fluid as in the case of a major burn (see **p 94**) or prolonged diarrhoea where fluid is drawn from the blood to make up.

3   The blood vessels may suddenly over-dilate (enlarge in diameter). This can be a toxic or allergic reaction to certain poisons or infections.

Whatever the cause, the result is a sudden big drop in blood pressure (circulatory collapse) and the casualty feels faint, giddy, nauseous and shivery. His skin is pale, cold and clammy. He may be panting and will have a weak pulse. If the shock is severe enough, the casualty will become drowsy, confused and eventually may lose consciousness altogether. Profound unrelieved shock leads to brain and kidney damage within a few minutes and, if prolonged, is fatal.

WHAT TO DO:

The aim of emergency aid is to try to improve the blood supply to the brain and other vital organs; to deal with any bleeding or other cause of the shock; and to get help fast.

1   If there is obvious serious bleeding, deal with it immediately (see **p 60**).

2   Send someone to call an ambulance (see **p 12**).

3   If the casualty is conscious, be cool, calm and reassuring.

4   If the casualty is conscious and you are certain that there is no spinal injury, lay him flat on his back and turn his head to one side in case he is sick. Do not put a pillow or anything under his head – the idea is to keep his head low in order to increase the blood supply to his brain. Instead, raise his legs above chest level (assuming that you have no reason to suspect a leg fracture) – this helps to push up the blood pressure a little.

5   Keep the casualty comfortable. Lay a coat or blanket over him, but **don't** let him get too warm because this will divert blood to the

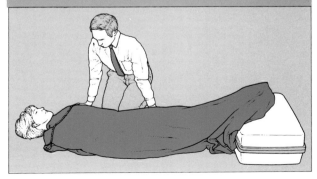

Keep a shocked casualty warm, his head low and his feet raised.

skin and further deprive vital organs. Loosen his collar to help him breathe. If he complains of thirst, moisten his lips with water but **don't** give him anything to drink as this increases the risk of him vomiting and may also prevent him being given an anaesthetic in hospital.

6   Keep checking the casualty's level of responsiveness every 10 minutes (see **p 16**).

7   If the casualty loses consciousness, open his airway and, if he keeps breathing, put him in the Recovery Position (see **p 22**). Check breathing and pulse every few minutes.

8   If the breathing or heart stops, begin resuscitation immediately (see **p 28** and **p 37**) and continue until medical help arrives.

HEART ATTACK:

Heart disease is the biggest single cause of sudden unexpected death in all 'developed' countries. Diet, smoking, lack of exercise and, possibly, stress all contribute to an epidemic which can kill people in the prime of life. Almost everyone reading this book is likely to know someone whose life has been ended prematurely by a killer which was virtually unknown 100 years ago.

There is often some confusion about terms: 'angina', 'heart attack' and 'cardiac arrest' all have different meanings.

Angina or Angina pectoris

The blood vessels leading to the heart have become permanently narrowed. Exercise or excitement may bring on pain in the chest and arms. Usually, resting brings immediate relief. Angina patients often carry pills containing glyceryl trinitrate which will dissolve quickly under the tongue. These relieve the pain. If the pain does not retreat after rest and after taking these pills, you should suspect the more serious problem of a heart attack.

Heart attack or coronary thrombosis

A clot of blood suddenly blocks a coronary artery which supplies blood to part of the heart. Without blood, the heart muscle cannot work properly, so the heart falters, causing the acute pain described as a 'heart attack'.

Cardiac arrest

The heart has stopped beating altogether. It may happen as the result of a heart attack, or may have some other cause such as electrocution. Either way, the casualty will be dead within a few minutes unless resuscitated.

Recognising a heart attack

There are two emergency first aid problems with a heart attack. One is recognising it for what it is; the other is knowing what to do.

We probably all think we are perfectly familiar with the symptoms of a heart attack. Characters in soap operas due for 'writing out' are frequently despatched by this means. In many an over-the-top adventure film the hero is saved from certain death by the scriptwriter giving the villain a coronary which causes him to clutch his chest and sink lifeless to the ground at the critical moment. Why then, when we are so familiar with the fiction, does it seem that so many of us do not know or recognise the symptoms in ourselves or others in real life? Here are two typical cases:

"

I woke up in the middle of the night with a bad pain in my chest. I'd been eating cheese for supper, and I put it down to indigestion. I felt rough the next day, but got to work somehow. That evening the same thing happened again. This time I thought I'd better call the doctor. He called an ambulance. The hospital were horrified when they found I'd been driving a heavy goods vehicle all day between the first attack and the second. I've had to retire early, but I consider myself lucky to be alive.

"

"

It was the worst pain I'd ever had – worse even than having a baby. Because I was so young – only forty-three – and female, the last thing in my mind was that it was a heart attack. I'd thought a heart attack meant a sudden stabbing pain in the middle of your chest. This pain gradually took over the whole of the upper part of my body, includ-

*ing my face, and I was sweating and naus-
eous. One of my colleagues insisted I went to
the office surgery and they whipped me off
to the hospital straight away. When I over-
heard them describing me as a 'cardiac case'
I was absolutely stunned. I'd thought I probably had food poisoning!* 〞

It is the first hour after an attack that is the most critical. At
the present time, certainly, many heart attack patients
present themselves for treatment late, sometimes too
late to be helped.

There are probably various reasons for this. One is that
the fictional treatment on television and in films or books
is often rather inaccurate and incomplete. Another is that,
in its first and mildest phases, a heart attack can indeed re-
semble other, less sinister conditions.

The symptoms

Most heart attack patients will experience some or all of
these symptoms:

- An uncomfortable feeling of overwhelming press-
  ure; gripping 'fullness' or pain in the centre of the
  chest.
- This pain spreading typically to arms, neck, throat,
  jaw and back.
- The pain developing over several minutes: it hardly
  ever starts abruptly.
- Feeling sick.
- Breathlessness.
- Severe giddiness or feeling of weakness.
- Pale skin, heavy sweating.
- Blue lips and finger tips.
- The casualty will often hold his chest and bend
  over.

Many heart attack patients will say, like the woman quoted above, that the pain is the worst they have ever experienced. But any chest pain accompanied by any of the other symptoms should be treated as a potential heart attack until proved otherwise.

One other point worth remembering is that many heart attack casualties will admit to several days of feeling over-whelmingly tired and decidedly unwell immediately before the critical phase of the illness. One, a school teacher who had his first (and only) attack at forty-two now describes it thus, fifteen years later:

"

It was at the end of the Christmas term. I was just dog tired for an entire week beforehand – not just the usual end-of-term tired – far, far worse. I was dragging myself around, and I had fairly frequent chest pains which didn't last very long. In the back of my mind I knew what it was. It didn't surprise me at all when I had the attack – I'd seen it coming really. **"**

This should not be taken to mean that everyone who feels tired and unwell is in line for a heart attack; this is most un-likely. Persistent tiredness is just one sign to be put with all the others.

Often the initial symptoms of a heart attack are fairly mild and people are reluctant to 'bother' the ambulance service or the hospitals. As one distinguished cardiologist said, 'Heaven is full of nice people who didn't want to bother their doctors.' The system is there to be used: don't hesitate if you are at all worried about someone's condition.

Because the family doctor is a more familiar figure, some people ring his or her number first. There are various reasons why this may not be the best action to take with a possible heart attack victim. Your doctor may not be able to provide full emergency cover: he or she may already be out on another call, and it may be several hours before they are able to visit you. Then, shocking as it may seem, very few doctors (GPs or otherwise) are actually trained in resuscitation as it is not usually a formal part of their training. If your casualty has a cardiac arrest, there is no guarantee that your doctor will have the up-to-date skills in cardio-pulmonary resuscitation (CPR) that are needed. However, as with all medical emergencies, you must use your own judgement. In a rural area where the ambulance is half an hour away, it may be much more sensible to call the local doctor than to wait.

Finally, it is most definitely not true that 'only a doctor' can call an ambulance to a heart attack victim. If you dial 999 and say that you suspect a heart attack, this is an official priority for the ambulance service.

You may need to take this action in spite of the patient's protests that he doesn't want to be a nuisance, that he must get on with his work, go home, or whatever. Over-rule all objections: it is better to be safe than sorry. This cautionary tale recounted to us by a BBC film crew member has a happy ending:

"

I was coming back from a long bout of film-ing. My colleague John (the junior electri-cian on the team) was driving. I began to feel ill – terrible pains on the chest and arm, feel-ing very sick, sweating and so on. John looked worried, but I just asked him to drop me off at home – I thought it was just an upset stomach. Fortunately, he'd done a first aid course and he recognised the symptoms. He said, 'I'm driving you straight to the hos-pital – you're an emergency. Don't worry – just relax.' I begged him not to – I was sure if I could get home to bed I'd be fine. He just ignored me and drove like the clappers – probably through several red lights – I don't remember. I passed out just as we got there. He quite definitely saved my life by being so insistent. I felt I owed it to him and to my doctors to reform my ways, so that was the end of smoking, drinking and overeating – I'm a reformed character!

99

WHAT TO DO:

1 **Get an ambulance.** The most important thing to do is to dial 999 and ask for an ambulance (see **p 12**). Tell ambulance control that you suspect a heart attack. ***Don't delay:*** remember that the first hour is vital. This is the period in which the person is most prone to cardiac arrest. If his heart does stop, the 'best' place for this to happen is in hospital where there are drugs and equipment available to help re-start the heart.

2 **Give reassurance.** Tell the patient that the ambulance is on its way. Speak calmly and quietly, and don't panic. Don't leave him, but don't 'fuss' him.

3 **Make the patient comfortable.** Let him choose a position in which he feels comfortable – usually half-sitting, half-lying, with knees bent. Don't let him walk about or go upstairs – this may put too much strain on the heart. Don't make the mistake of fiddling officiously with his clothing. Ask first, and only loosen clothes if they are obviously tight or uncomfortable.

Don't give him anything to eat or drink; this will only increase the feeling of nausea and if he loses consciousness and vomits he may inhale his vomit and choke (see **p 19**).

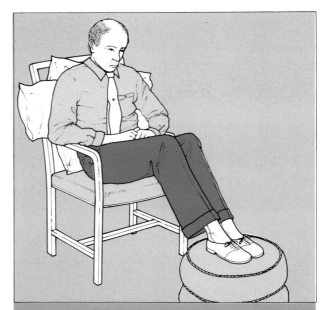

Whilst waiting for the ambulance most heart-attack victims find a half-sitting, half-lying position with their knees bent most comfortable. Don't let them walk around or eat or drink.

4 **Keep checking his level of consciousness.** As long as he is still conscious, there is nothing more you can do until the ambulance arrives except to continue calmly offering reassurance.

5 **If he becomes unconscious** (i.e. cannot be roused) but is still breathing, put him in the Recovery Position (see **p 22**) and keep checking his breathing.

6 **If the breathing and pulse stop.** Begin resuscitation and don't give up. Your aim is to keep his circulation going at least enough to prevent brain damage until medical help arrives (see **pp 27–44**).

These are the basic guidelines, but circumstances in real life often make it difficult to follow them to the letter. You should remember, too, that if you have to give resuscitation and fail, you have no way of knowing at the time how much the patient has already been damaged beyond recovery, as in the following case:

> **"**
> *My husband had a sudden massive coronary one night just as he was climbing into bed. He collapsed between the bed and the wall. He was a big man, and I am quite severely disabled myself. I just couldn't move him to the floor – he was jammed. To this day I torture myself with 'if only' thoughts, even though the coroner was extremely kind and sympathetic. He said that so much of my husband's heart muscle had been destroyed that he could never have recovered, even if I'd been able to attempt first aid.*
> **"**

Sometimes, however, in spite of very difficult circumstances, it *is* just possible to give sufficient help to save life. One of the first 'rescues' which emerged from the 'Save A Life' campaign involved just such an event:

> **"**
> *A bus driver in Essex collapsed at the wheel of his one-man bus. Two women passengers came to his aid in spite of the fact that he had fallen very awkwardly into the gangway of the bus. One of his rescuers was pregnant, and the other had never done a first aid course – she had simply watched the television programmes. Nonetheless they succeeded in reviving him: one gave him mouth-to-mouth resuscitation while the other did chest compressions.*
> **"**

This story proves again that resuscitation in heart attack cases can be effective, even when it is not done 'by the book'. When we first showed the 'Save A Life' pro- grammes to groups of experts up and down the country at preview meetings, some of them were mildly critical of this lack of textbook perfection in the real-life stories fea- tured in the programmes. The following example, in par- ticular, was the subject of some debate:

66

> My mother called me in the middle of the night to say that my father was ill. I went into their room and he was lying on his side very awkwardly. He is a heavy man and I had a ter- rible job turning him on to his back. He looked blue. I tried to check his pulse in his wrist but couldn't find it; I tried his neck but still couldn't find any pulse. I looked at his chest to see if he was breathing and he wasn't; his eyes were 'in the back of his head'. I put his head back and started the mouth-to-mouth and chest massage, watch- ing his chest to see if it was rising and falling – it seemed like ages, but it was probably only a few minutes before he gave a huge sigh and I thought, 'That's either the last breath coming out, or mine going in.' Then suddenly he was one big bath of sweat. His eyes came down and he groaned, came round and said he thought he was having a nightmare . . . and that was it.

99

The experts were worried by the fact that the rescuer in this story had not put her father on the floor – a bouncy, unresistant bed is not the ideal surface for chest com- pressions. They also commented that her account of her actions shows that they were not in the 'perfect' sequence of the first aid manuals.

This was all absolutely true. However, the reality was that the practical difficulties of turning her father from his side on to his back in itself almost defeated her, let alone the 'ideal' of transferring him to the harder surface of the floor in a small bedroom, a manoeuvre which would have taken several more precious minutes. Above all, the indisputable fact is that her father is still alive and well several years later, whereas without her help he would certainly have died.

Avoiding a heart attack

Heart disease is mostly preventable. The rules for prudent living and a healthy heart are:

Smoking: Avoid it altogether. Stopping smoking is the best thing you can do for your heart.

Food: Choose a diet low in animal fat and salt, but high in fibre, fresh fruit and vegetables.

Weight: Keep your weight within the sensible limits for your height.

Alcohol: Drink moderately – no more than 35 'single' drinks (i.e. equivalent to half a pint of bitter) a week for men, 21 for women.

Exercise: Take regular, sustained, moderately vigorous exercise – say, 20 to 30 minutes two or three times a week.

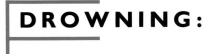

DROWNING:

Drowning is the third most common cause of accidental death: about 800 people die this way every year. Some of them are strong adult swimmers who get into sudden difficulty in the sea; some are young people fooling about on canal or river banks; some are toddlers who drown in very shallow water in a garden pond or even a bath.

Most of these deaths arise from accidents that were preventable in the first place. But, equally importantly, a rescuer's prompt action and willingness to 'have a go' can save many lives that would otherwise be lost. The majority of victims of near-drowning are fit young people who stand every chance of making a complete recovery if breathing and heart are re-started quickly.

Two important don'ts

1 DON'T leap unthinkingly to the rescue. Your first priority must be your own safety. Many heroic would-be rescuers put their own lives at risk because they do not think carefully about the circumstances.

Remember:

- Sea, river or canal water will be cold, probably murky; you may not know how deep it is. There may be strong currents that could sweep both you and the original victim away.

- Clothes will make swimming more difficult.

- The victim will probably be panicking and thrashing about. He could strike you or pull you under.

- A swimming rescue is difficult unless you are a trained and competent life-saver.

- Most drownings happen only a few metres from dry land. Most victims can swim. Keep on dry land yourself whenever possible; throw a rope, pole or lifebuoy, or hold out an arm. Lie down on the bank so that you will not be pulled in yourself.

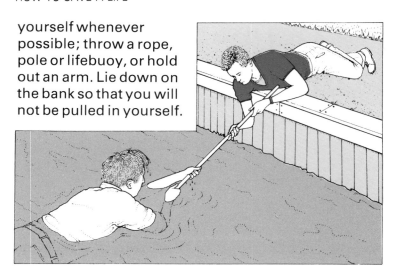

2   DON'T waste time trying to empty water from the casualty's lungs. It is a myth that this is necessary.

● In some drownings, the throat closes up as a reaction to the water, so there is no water in the lungs anyway.

● Even if the lungs do contain water, there will be enough spare capacity to allow air to get in or out.

● Trying to 'empty' the lungs wastes precious time which should be spent on resuscitation.

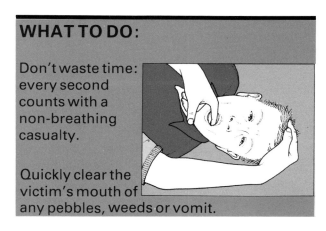

WHAT TO DO:

Don't waste time: every second counts with a non-breathing casualty.

1   Quickly clear the victim's mouth of any pebbles, weeds or vomit.

2 Start resuscitation immediately. Begin by opening the airway and giving mouth-to-mouth breathing in the water if necessary.

3 Continue on dry land with the full ABC: open the casualty's airway, give mouth-to-mouth breathing and chest compressions.

4 As soon as possible, send someone to call an ambulance.

5 The casualty is likely to have froth round his mouth. He may also vomit. Be prepared to continue in spite of this until breathing is restored.

6 If the casualty is breathing but remains unconscious, put him in the Recovery Position (see **p 22**).

7 Warm up the casualty. Someone who has nearly drowned will normally be cold and is at risk from hypothermia. Try to prevent further dangerous loss of body heat while you are waiting for the ambulance. Cover the casualty lightly with blankets or put him in a warm bath.

8 Get the casualty into hospital. Anyone rescued from drowning must go to hospital for observation. Water drawn into the lungs affects the way in which oxygen is transferred to the blood and there is considerable danger of what is called 'secondary drowning' for anything up to 72 hours later. The casualty's lungs fill with fluid from his own body and his life is endangered again unless prompt medical help is given. So, however fit and well the casualty appears, always call an ambulance and always insist that he goes to hospital.

Weighing up the risks

Rescues from drowning often involve considerable heroism on the part of the rescuer. No one case will be exactly like another, but the circumstances of real life are frequently more complex than the first aid manuals suggest. One widely reported recent rescue involved a family of five whose car skidded at night on black ice and somersaulted into a pond. Someone living in a cottage a few yards away heard a thud followed by the noise of his ducks quacking. He rushed out with a torch and saw the car upside down in the water. He recalls:

"

I waded into the water and one by one pulled out three adults and a little boy. The mother was screaming, 'My baby, my baby!', so I waded in again. I lost my torch in all the confusion, but I searched the car until I found a fluffy bundle. I couldn't undo her safety strap, but the baby's father plunged back into the water and between us we pulled the child out. By this time another neighbour had arrived. The baby was blue and apparently dead. My neighbour had turned up by then. He is a farmer, and he decided he must treat her like a breech-birth calf, so he tipped her upside down, pinched her nose and gave her the kiss of life and chest compressions. The baby started to breathe. By this time the police had come, and a police constable wrapped her in tin foil, then put her in a warm bath in our house, by which time the ambulance had arrived. She was kept in hospital for a bit, but she was completely OK when they released her. The silly thing is that I can't swim, but I knew the pond was only about 4 feet deep. It was icy cold, very dark and very frightening, but I felt all the time that between us we could do it.

"

This rescue is perhaps less risky to a non-swimming rescuer than it first appears when you remember that the person knew how deep the pond was and that help was at hand. The prompt action of his neighbour re-started the baby's heart and breathing, and the policeman's knowledge of how to prevent hypothermia meant that there was a good chance of a successful rescue.

Sadly, the circumstances are not always so favourable and many rescues, like the one described below, do fail:

❝

I was messing about having a great time in the river with my brother. We saw this lady swimming on the other side and she seemed to be all right. Then suddenly she gave a yell and sank out of sight. We didn't know what to do, but she didn't come up again so we dived after her. For years afterwards I had nightmares about the dark mud and weeds. It took ages to find her because the river was so dirty that we couldn't see. She kept slipping out of our grasp. Finally we got her out. We were covered in mud and weeds and so was she. We did our best and worked on her for ages – we knew what to do because of a Royal Life Saving Society course. She vomited at one stage and we thought she'd be OK. Someone else had called an ambulance, but she was dead on arrival at the hospital. We felt terrible, but I think she'd just been in the water too long.

❞

When do you stop?

It is vital that you carry on attempting resuscitation either until the casualty is breathing unaided again, or until medical help arrives. Even if the casualty has been in the water for a long time, it is still worth trying to resuscitate him and continuing for as long as your energy holds. David Bunch, a lifeguard on Brighton Beach, describes his experience of such a case:

"

Someone said a young girl was in the water. I dived in and pulled her out – she was obviously 'dead' and she could have been in the water for some time. I cleared her mouth of shingle and lay her on the beach, scooping out a place for her head to help with opening her airway. I gave her CPR for twenty minutes, and for a long time there was no sign of life, but finally she gave a gasp, then I felt a pulse. She made a full recovery. **"**

Continuing resuscitation for a long time is often essential when medical help is a long way off, as in this incident.

"

When a diver, who got caught up in a rope at a depth of 20 metres off the Cornish coast and lost his breathing mouthpiece, was found by his two companions, he was unconscious. They cut him free and got him to the surface and onto the boat, but by this time he was not breathing and had no pulse. Frothy blood was coming out of his mouth.

Another companion, who was trained in life-saving, took over and, with help, gave mouth-to-mouth breathing and chest compressions. Meanwhile the skipper called up the lifeboat on the ship-to-shore radio.

After about 20 minutes the diver began to breathe again unaided, and when the lifeboat arrived some 45 minutes later he was conscious. 'My wife will kill me when she finds out about this!' he said. Thanks to his friends' prompt action, he made a full recovery. **"**

It seems that some humans, particularly young children, demonstrate the 'mammalian diving reflex' when immersed in cold water. This means that their bodies respond to the emergency by almost shutting down the oxygen supply to every part except the heart and the brain.

Avoiding trouble

Observe a few simple rules:

- Learn to swim.
- Don't go into the water alone.
- Swim only at supervised sites: pools and beaches where there is a lifeguard on duty.
- Don't dive into shallow water or water where you don't know the depth.
- Overconfidence is the swimmer's worst enemy. Stop well before tiredness affects your judgement.
- Don't let children play unsupervised in or near water; even a garden pond can be lethal.
- Alcohol impairs judgement. Don't drink before swimming. In roughly one quarter of drownings, the victim has been drinking.

CHOKING:

" We were out to celebrate my daughter's birthday. During the meal someone made me laugh and I began to choke. One guest, a nurse for several years, handed me a glass of water; a pharmacist friend just sat and stared; my husband gently rubbed my back. I began to get very frightened as I could not breathe. My seventeen-year-old son jumped up from his seat, stood me up and gave me the 'bear hug' treatment – he had to do it three times! What a relief – I thought my end had come. Paul had been through the Duke of Edinburgh course on first aid. Thank God he recalled what he had been taught and put it into action. **"**

The viewer quoted above, who wrote in from Lincoln after seeing the 'Save A Life' television programme on choking, vividly describes the terror and helplessness that the choking casualty feels. The setting, too, is typical: a family celebration with perhaps a glass or two of wine (alcohol interferes with the swallowing reflex), the ineffectual reaction of other bystanders, the dramatic relief when the obstruction is removed.

A death from choking is nearly always an avoidable tragedy. The victim has died from a straightforward sudden obstruction to breathing and most often – in perhaps nine cases out of ten – the death is unnecessary: if someone present had known what to do, it could have been prevented. Unlike in cases of heart attack, there is no underlying disease predisposing the victim to disaster. As soon as the casualty can breathe again, he or she makes a complete and uneventful recovery.

In the USA, where death from choking is more common than here, it is often described as a 'café coronary'. The reason is that the symptoms can at first glance look like a sudden heart attack. A large piece of food blocks the airway completely, the victim cannot speak, becomes blue, falls unconscious and dies before anyone realises what is happening.

Death from choking can also occur when people drink too much, overdose on drugs or both. Some of these cases make headlines, but there are many dozens of others yearly where the inquest report occupies only a few lines in the local paper: for instance, that of the young postman in Brighton who drank a bottle of vodka for a bet and was found dead in bed next morning. He had choked to death on his own vomit.

The classic choking incident, however, happens in public and frequently bystanders do not realise how serious it is, as in the following example:

“

My mother-in-law was staying with us for Christmas and we were all laughing and joking with the children. She handed round some boiled sweets and took one herself. Within seconds she was gasping and clutching her throat. My husband thought she was just fooling about and went on laughing. Fortunately I'd done a 'lifesaver' course and I realised that she was choking because she was turning blue. I got behind her and did the Heimlich [see page 87] two or three times: the sweet came out like a cork out of a bottle and she was fine, though upset. Even after that my husband thought it was a joke. He soon sobered up when he realised what could have happened.

”

85

Sometimes the victim feels so embarrassed at making a display that he or she rushes off to the lavatory and locks the door – which is extremely dangerous.

WHAT TO DO:

1 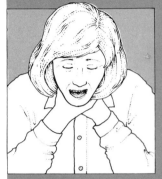 Recognise choking for what it is: a serious emergency which can cause death within minutes. The choking casualty will usually clutch her neck, may wheeze or gasp, and will begin turning blue. The veins at the side of the neck may stand out.

2 Don't let her lock herself in the lavatory. Social embarrassment is preferable to death!

3 Encourage her to make coughing motions – this may help. Reassure her and stay calm.

4 If this fails, bend her right over so that her head is lower than her lungs: gravity will help dislodge the object.

5 Strike her sharply between the shoulder blades three or four times, using the heel of your hand. This should not be a 'pat' – it should be a blow, hard enough to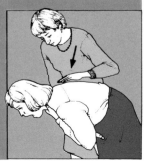

feel uncomfortable and strong enough to force out the object.

6 *If this fails, as a last resort, you should try the Heimlich manoeuvre (also called the 'abdominal thrust').*

The Heimlich manoeuvre

Stand behind the casualty and clench one fist, thumb facing inwards towards her stomach. Grab this fist with your other hand. One fist should be under the ribs, between the navel and breastbone. Now pull sharply inwards and upwards, three or four times. You are pushing the upper abdomen against the lungs with the aim of forcing air violently upwards.

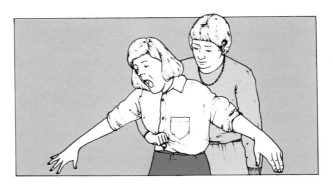

The Heimlich manoeuvre

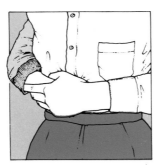
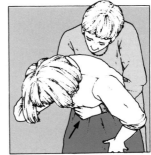

We have suggested using the Heimlich manoeuvre as a last resort because this is currently advised by the three British voluntary societies concerned with first aid (the Red Cross, St John Ambulance and St Andrew's Ambulance Association). The American view is different, however. The American Heart Association now recommends that the Heimlich manoeuvre is used first because it considers it to be more effective. In one bizarre experiment where heroic volunteers were asked to choke deliberately (the obstruction was securely tied to a piece of thread), the outcome seemed to be that backslaps tended to drive the object further down the throat, whereas the Heimlich manoeuvre was usually successful.

But the British view is that the Heimlich manoeuvre is risky because, theoretically, there is a danger of damaging the liver and the gullet. However, there is certainly now plenty of anecdotal evidence that it works. Faced with a friend or member of your family who might otherwise die, you should not hesitate to try the Heimlich manoeuvre. Be warned, though, that this is one technique to learn properly under supervision with a trained instructor. Don't try it out 'for a practice'. Even in classes it is usually demonstrated only by one experienced tutor on another.

What if the casualty is unconscious?

1 Send someone to call an ambulance.

2 Place her on the floor and try to sweep out any visible object with a bent finger.

3 If this fails, roll the casualty on to her side and try back blows.

4 If there is still no response, roll her on to her back and kneel astride her. Put the heel of one hand in the centre of the abdomen between the navel and breastbone, and cover it with the other hand. Keep your elbows straight.

5 Press inwards and upwards sharply and firmly three or four times (see illustration opposite).

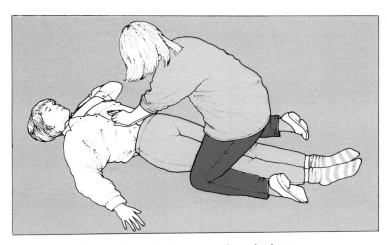

Abdominal thrusts for a choking casualty who loses consciousness.

6   If there is still no success, attempt mouth-to-mouth breathing. If her pulse has stopped, give chest compressions. It is possible that there may be a very narrow passage in the airway, or that the object may have moved down into the chest.

7   Keep doing this as a sequence: that is, back blows, followed by abdominal thrusts, then CPR. Don't give up until medical help arrives.

Children

Anyone who is a parent will know that the main way in which very young children explore the world is through their mouths. Every new object is automatically tasted. When it is a very small object, the result can be that the child chokes, as one mother's story illustrates:

66

My youngest child was only six months old when this happened. The older children had been playing marbles and they'd left them all over the floor. I was tidying up in the kitchen and I'd left the baby on the carpet in the dining room. I thought she was quite safe just sitting there with a few toys as I believed she was a long way from crawling. My back was turned only for a second, but when I looked round she was crawling or lunging towards a marble. It was like watching a film in slow motion – I saw her take it and put it into her mouth. My running towards her must have startled her because she got it stuck in her throat. I just instinctively held her upside down and smacked her hard between the shoulders. The marble came shooting out. We both cried afterwards – she with indignation, I with relief – and guilt that I'd let it happen!

99

WHAT TO DO:

If a child chokes, the treatment is the same as for an adult, but you must use much less force.

For a baby

1   Lay the baby along your arm, head pointing well down. Smack her sharply between the shoulder blades (see opposite). In the great majority of cases this will be enough to dislodge an object stuck in the throat.

2   If back slaps fail, lay the baby on a firm surface and open her airway. Place two fingers between her navel and breastbone and press quickly with an upwards and forwards movement three or four times (see illustration opposite).

For a toddler

1   Sit in a chair and lay the toddler over your knee, head pointing well down. Slap her four times between her shoulders.

2   If this fails, you should try a modified form of the Heimlich manoeuvre (see **p 87**). Sit the child on your lap, with her back against your stomach. Clench your fist and place it, thumb inwards, just under her ribs. Grasp this hand with your other hand and press inwards and upwards three or four times, but not so fiercely as with an adult.

For an older child

Treat an older child in the same way as an adult, but use less pressure according to the child's age, height and weight.

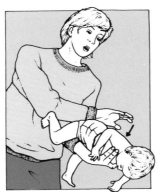

Back slaps for a baby.

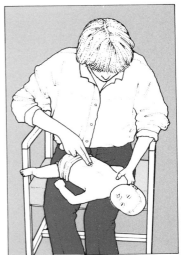

Abdominal thrusts for a baby. Use only if all else fails.

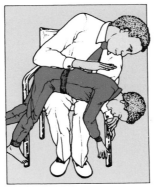

Back slaps for a toddler.

Avoiding choking

Prevention is better than cure. Always follow these guidelines:

1 Cut food up into small pieces.

2 Chew food thoroughly, especially if you wear dentures.

3 Avoid laughing and talking while you still have food in your mouth.

4 Don't let babies and toddlers play with toys that have small components – tiny Lego pieces, marbles, pull-rings from drink cans and beads can all be lethal. So, too, can nuts – peanuts can be specially dangerous as they are easily inhaled and can lodge in the lungs: don't let young children eat them. Boiled sweets are unsuitable for children under four.

5 If you suspect that your partner or teenage child has been drinking heavily and/or taking drugs and he has fallen into a deep sleep, turn him into the Recovery Position (see **p 22**) to sleep it off and keep monitoring him through the night. Don't let him sleep on his back.

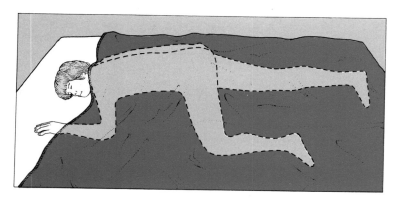

BURNS AND SCALDS:

> **"** We had invited my parents around for tea, and because I was showing off I'd put a tablecloth out – something we normally never do. We were just sitting down and getting everybody settled when our eighteen-month-old son seized the edge of the cloth and pulled the teapot full of scalding hot water all over his shoulder and arm. My mother-in-law was flapping about shouting, 'Get some butter!', but I was super-calm. I'd done a first aid badge at Guides, and I clearly remembered what to do. I just picked him up and flung him into the sink, clothes and all, and drenched the arm in cold water. He was yelling his head off – a high-pitched scream, really – but I kept the tap running, then peeled off his shirt. Within about ten minutes the skin had cooled down and looked a lot less red. I covered it with a bandage and I did take him to the doctor, but he didn't need treatment. I'm sure that was thanks to the fact that I knew what to do and didn't panic. **"**

As this example shows, human skin is amazingly tough and resilient stuff, but if it is seriously damaged by a burn from fire, boiling liquid, electrical current or chemicals, life can be at risk. Why?

- In a severe burn, so much fluid may leak from the circulatory system that shock may develop. A badly shocked casualty may die (see **p 64**).

• Normally the skin protects us from bacterial infection. A seriously burned area will have lost its ability to keep bacteria at bay.

• A burn or scald affecting the face may produce swelling in the throat which could close up the airway and cause suffocation.

• Some burns involve chemicals which not only affect the skin but also spread to other organs of the body where they may do considerable damage.

Minor burns are part and parcel of everyday living and are simple to treat by holding the burn under a slowly running cold tap for ten minutes or so. This cools the skin down and usually provides instant relief.

We are concerned here with the kind of serious burn which is a real emergency needing prompt action and medical help.

When is a burn 'serious'?

• When the area affected is larger than 1 square inch. The bigger the burnt area, the greater the danger of infection and shock.

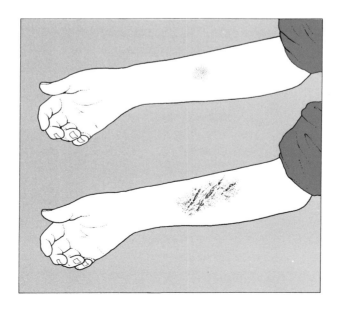

- When the burn does not hurt. A deep burn destroys the nerve endings in the skin.
- When the skin looks pale, waxy or charred: this also indicates a deep burn.
- When the casualty shows all the classic signs of shock (see **p 64**): feeling faint, sick, cold and clammy, with shallow rapid breathing.
- If the casualty becomes unconscious.
- When a burn is associated with electric shock.
- When a burn or scald has affected the throat or mouth.

For many years mythology abounded regarding the home treatment of burns, much of it dangerously wrong. The guidelines below should dispel any misconceptions:

DON'T cover a burn with butter or any kind of ointment. It will not help to cool the skin down and may introduce infection.

DON'T put on a sticking plaster because it may be impossible to remove later without damaging the skin even more. Similarly, don't put on cotton wool.

DON'T break any blisters as they are offering a fragile protection to the skin underneath. Breaking them opens the burn to infection.

DON'T pull away dry, charred clothing as, again, you may damage the skin underneath.

WHAT TO DO:

1 **If clothing is on fire:** Put the flames out by starving them of oxygen. You can do this in two ways – choose whichever is quicker:
   - Either douse the flames with water from a bowl or bucket, or wrap the casualty tightly in a coat or blanket. Don't use anything made of nylon fabric to smother the flames as it burns easily, melts, and will make matters worse.

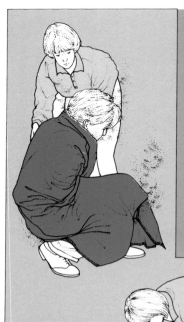

- Lay him down quickly. A standing casualty offers an upwards path to the flames. Laying him down will help put them out.
- Don't roll him on the floor as this may spread the flames rather than put them out.

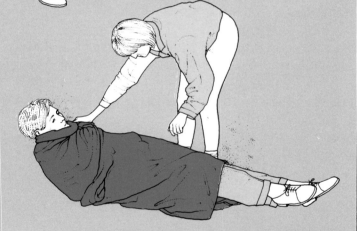

- Soak the burnt clothes in cold water. This will stop them smouldering and will also help to cool the burnt area of skin beneath.

2   Offer reassurance and comfort. The great majority of burns victims are children and elderly people. It is important to prevent further panic by staying calm yourself.

3 Burnt skin swells, but the swelling becomes more pronounced as the minutes pass. Remove any rings, watches, bracelets or anything constricting before the swelling starts: they may be much more difficult to take off later.

4 A scald often involves clothing: for instance, in the case of a toddler who spills the contents of a hot teapot over her arm. Cover the affected area in cold water, then gently remove the clothes.

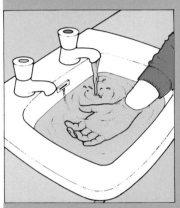

5 For chemical burns, flood the area with cold running water and gently remove any affected clothing, making sure that you do not contaminate yourself while doing so. If possible use a shower, hose or bucket.

6 Cover the burn as soon as possible to prevent infection. Ideally you should use a proper sterile dressing, but it may be impossible to find one that is the right size and easily available. If so, don't waste time – use any non-fluffy clean material: a handkerchief, a pillowcase or sheet, or a linen tea-towel can all be used successfully. Secure it in place with a bandage, safety pin, tie or scarf or, failing these, hold it there yourself. It is useful to know that, in kitchen accidents

involving burns, plastic cling film makes an ideal improvised dressing. It clings to the skin without sticking and can be wound round a limb or the chest so that it stays put.

7   Assume that the casualty is shocked; raise her legs above chest level and cover her lightly with something warm.

8   If she is conscious, let her have occasional sips of cold water to replace lost fluid.

9   Monitor her breathing and heartbeat. If she becomes unconscious, put her in the Recovery Position (see **p 22**). Be prepared to resuscitate if necessary.

10   Telephone for medical help.

Safety Precautions

Cookers

Cookers easily top the list as causes of fires and burns. Smoking fat or oil in a chip pan will ignite on its own if left to continue heating up. When you can see smoke coming from a pan, turn off the heat immediately *without moving the pan*.

Never leave a pan of hot fat or oil unattended. Never fill a pan to more than one third of its capacity with fat or oil. If the worst happens and the pan catches fire:

- Turn off the heat.

- Leave the pan where it is. Moving it will fan the flames and you may burn your hands and face.

- Smother the flames with a damp teatowel or a large lid. If you have one, a fire blanket is the most effective way of preventing the fire spreading further. Don't throw water on the burning fat: this will make the flames worse.

- Leave the pan undisturbed for at least thirty minutes after you have put out the fire.

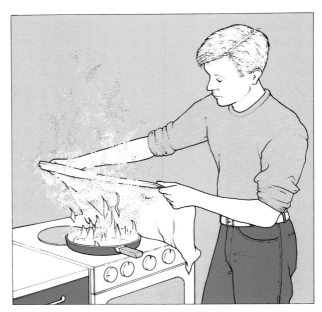

If a cooking pan catches fire, cover it quickly with a damp tea towel. Don't move the pan for 30 minutes.

Heaters

Heaters are responsible for about 5000 serious accidents a year. Observing some simple safety rules reduces the risks considerably:

● Don't try to dry or air clothes too near a radiant electric fire or oil heater.

● Keep heaters away from curtains and furniture.

● Never move or fill a lit paraffin heater.

● Choose the position of a paraffin heater carefully. It should be in the place where it is least likely to get knocked over by a swinging door, by children or pets.

Open fires

If you have young children or elderly people in the household, always use a fireguard that covers the entire fireplace, and make sure that it is in place last thing at night. Don't put a mirror over the fireplace as this encourages people to go too close to the fire.

Furniture and clothing

Modern upholstered furniture is often filled with materials which give off highly toxic fumes when they burn. These fumes can be lethal within two or three minutes. Such fires often start very slowly. For instance, a lighted cigarette can smoulder unnoticed for many hours if it has rolled down between the seat and arm of a chair. If you are buying new upholstered furniture, look for the tag that will tell you what the filling is. Choose flame-retardant materials whenever possible.

Pyjamas are safer for children and old people than nightdresses (though children's nightdresses must, by law, be made of flame-retardant material).

Smokers

People who smoke are potentially a fire hazard. People who smoke in bed are a particular risk as they can easily (and often do) fall asleep with a lighted cigarette in their hand, thus setting fire to their bed. If you smoke, or have a smoker in your household, try to keep these rules:

- Hide matches and lighters from children.
- Don't ever smoke in bed.
- Have plenty of ashtrays available.
- Make sure that discarded cigarettes in an ashtray are properly put out before you empty it.

Electrical Safety

Electrical fires and accidents are usually the result of overloading a circuit, or caused by a fault which has developed in an old wiring system.

- Always switch off and unplug appliances that are not in use. This is especially important with television sets and computers.
- Any wiring system more than 25 years old needs checking. Electricity Boards will do this free of charge.
- Try to avoid using adaptors and thus overloading one socket. Have extra sockets installed instead.

● Use the correct fuse for each appliance and the correct wattage of light bulb for a lamp. Don't cover a lampshade with paper or fabric – it may catch fire.

● Don't take electric heaters into a bathroom. Have a safe wall heater fitted instead.

● Don't handle any electrical appliance with wet hands.

If an electrical appliance (other than a computer or television set) does catch fire, this is what to do:

● Switch off the power at the mains.

● Unplug the affected appliance.

● Now that the power is switched off, you can extinguish the fire with water.

In the case of fire starting in a computer or television set:

● Switch off the power at your main fuse box.

● Throw a blanket or coat over the appliance; the reason for this different treatment is that there may still be some residual electricity in the set.

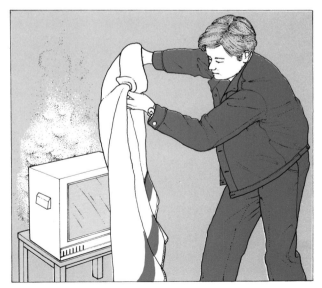

If your television catches fire, switch off the power at the mains and cover the set with a blanket. Do NOT touch the plug.

ELECTRIC SHOCK:

We all know that electricity is a powerful but dangerous friend. Some electrical accidents are minor – a mild shock and nothing more. But if electricity is out of control because say, an iron flex is badly damaged, or a faulty switch is touched with wet hands, the results can be fatal. The electric current may leave deep burns both where it enters and leaves the body. As it passes through, it may even make the heart stop, or affect the part of the brain that controls breathing.

WHAT TO DO:

Beware of becoming part of the accident yourself. Don't touch the casualty until you are sure that he is no longer in contact with the current.

1   Switch off the power at the socket and pull the plug out. If for some reason this is impossible, switch it off at the main fuse box.

2   If you cannot switch off the power at all, push the casualty away from the source of current by using a broom handle, a dining chair, a stool or some other means of levering him to safety, which does not involve your touching him. Alternatively, tow him away with a looped scarf or the hook of a walking stick or umbrella. Stand on something which will insulate you – for instance, a dry folded towel, a wad of dry newspaper or a rubber mat.

3   Check the casualty's breathing and heart-beat. If he is unconscious but breathing, put him in the Recovery Position (see **p 22**). Be prepared to resuscitate the casualty if his breathing and heart have stopped.

4   Cover the burn with a clean dressing (see **p 97**).

5   Treat a conscious casualty for shock (see **p 65**).

6   Call an ambulance. Anyone who has had a serious electric shock must go to hospital: the burns may be more severe than they look. It is also possible that the victim's heart may have been affected by the incident and he will certainly need to be under medical observation for a while.

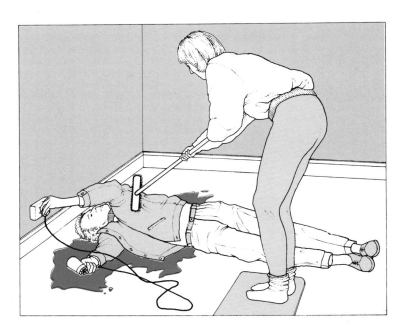

Do not touch the casualty if the electricity is still on. Use a broom handle or wooden chair to push him clear of the power source.

High-voltage emergencies

Any accident involving overhead power cables (for instance at pylons, railway lines and on some industrial sites) is extremely dangerous to bystanders. These sources can give a fatal shock at up to 18 metres (20 yards). **DON'T APPROACH** unless you are certain that the power supply has been turned off.

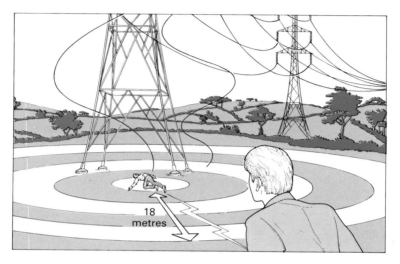

POISONING:

" *I came home to find my flat mate sprawled face down on the bed. She looked blue and there was an empty bottle of pills on the bed. She was just about still breathing. I called an ambulance immediately – there was nothing more I could do except give the bottle of pills to the ambulance man. Unfortunately, she died on the way to hospital. I have reproached myself ever since, wondering what more I might have done, even though I knew rationally, that I did everything possible.* **"**

Our environment is full of poisons, many of them friendly, useful products if correctly employed, yet deadly if carelessly used. Household bleach is harmless enough when it is killing all known germs in the lavatory, but it becomes a lethal liquid if swallowed by a toddler who thinks that, because it comes in a bottle, it must be drinkable. Alcohol has its place as a socially acceptable drug, but it too is a poison. Prescribed drugs may be used by intending suicides; illegally acquired drugs are bought and sold everywhere and accidental overdoses are common. Chemicals may be accidentally inhaled or absorbed from industrial pollution; and car or lorry drivers can be poisoned by carbon monoxide from a faulty exhaust. And as if that weren't enough, there are also all the natural hazards: poisonous plants, animals and insects. But, whatever the cause, there are some simple steps you can take to help a victim of poisoning.

WHAT TO DO:

1 **Assess the scene.** Usually, it is obvious
what has happened. A conscious casualty
will be able to tell you; there may be bottles
of pills or containers of other sorts lying
around. With inhaled poisons like gases, the
smell will tell you all you need to know.

2 **Separate the casualty from the poison if
necessary,** but take care yourself. For
instance, do not contaminate yourself with
dangerous chemicals; don't enter a gas-or
smoke-filled room unless you are sure that
you can get out again quickly.

3 **Assess the casualty's symptoms.** Poisons
produce different reactions which may
include shock (see **p 64**), convulsions, burns
around the mouth or on the skin, vomiting
and unconsciousness.

4 **Check the casualty's breathing and pulse.**
Put an unconscious casualty in the Recovery
Position (see **p 22**). Be prepared to resusci-
tate.

5 **Dial 999 and get help fast.**

6 **Don't encourage the casualty to be sick:**
this may do more harm than good. In cases
where the victim has swallowed a corrosive
poison, such as bleach, ammonia, washing
soda, drain cleaner, paint stripper, dish-
washer detergent or petrol, which may
leave burns around the mouth, it is even
more important that you don't encourage
vomiting. Being sick will damage the casualty's throat and mouth even more by bring-
ing them into contact with the poison again.

Instead, give the casualty water or milk to drink. The idea is to dilute the poison in the stomach.

7   Don't give mouth-to-mouth resuscitation to a victim with burns around the mouth, as you could become contaminated yourself. Mouth-to-nose might be possible, if you can close the victim's mouth and cover it with something impervious such as a plastic bag.

8   When the ambulance arrives, tell the crew what you have seen and done. Give them any pills, bottles or other containers which you think may have been the source of the poison. The hospital will also find it useful to have a sample of vomit.

Preventing poisoning

● Never store weedkillers or substances like paint thinners in bottles or containers other than the ones in which they were bought.

● Store household and garden chemicals carefully in places where children cannot reach them.

● Invest in a lockable medicine cabinet and store all drugs inside it. Don't leave drugs or medicine lying about where children can find them.

UNCONSCIOUSNESS:

As we have said, unconsciousness is in itself potentially life-threatening because an unconscious casualty left lying on her back can suffocate on her own
tongue. In most cases you don't need to concern
yourself too much about the cause of the unconsciousness: it is more important to open her airway
(see **p 18**), to turn her into the Recovery Position (see
p 22), to keep checking breathing and pulse, and to be
ready to start resuscitation if necessary.

People do often ask, though, about particular conditions which can cause unconsciousness, so we
have included brief details of how to manage the
most common of them – diabetic coma (**p 109**), stroke
(**p 111**), epileptic fit (**p 113**), hypothermia (**p 116**) and
overdose (**p 105**).

There are a number of levels of responsiveness (or
lack of it) through which a casualty goes, from being
fully conscious to being deeply unconscious:

1 **Fully conscious** – responds normally to conver-
   sation.

2 **Drowsy** – responds only to direct questions.

3 **Confused** – responds inaccurately to simple
   questions.

4 **Semi-conscious** – responds only to simple com-
   mands.

5 **Unconscious** – responds only to pain (e.g. pinched
   skin).

6 **Deeply unconscious** – does not respond to anything.

A casualty who is semi-conscious or unconscious
should be assessed and treated according to the
sequence laid out on **pp 16–17**.

DIABETIC EMERGENCY:

In diabetes, the body has lost its ability to control the level of sugar in the blood. Most of the time, diabetics can manage their condition well by dietary control or insulin injections, or both, but sometimes they get a sudden surge or drop in blood sugar. Too much either way can produce unconsciousness and, if untreated, death.

Too much sugar:

This condition usually builds up slowly. The victim will probably recognise its onset and will call for help. He may be drowsy and his breath may smell of pear drops. There is nothing you can do to help him except to get him to hospital fast. If he becomes unconscious, turn him into the Recovery Position (see **p 22**).

Too little sugar:

It is much more common for this condition to overtake a diabetic suddenly. The problem for a bystander is usually recognising it, as the following case illustrates:

"

I was waiting for a bus when I saw a middle-aged man lurching round, then keeling over. Because of the kind of area it was – full of drunks and vagrants – no one took a scrap of notice. He was carrying a briefcase, a bit unlikely for a tramp! I ran over to him, thinking he might be having a heart attack. He looked very sweaty and pale, and kept fumbling in his jacket and mumbling something. It suddenly struck me that he might be a diabetic so I felt for his wallet and looked inside. Sure enough there was a diabetic ID card. There was quite a little crowd round him by now, so I sent a young chap off to the snack bar for some warm tea with masses of sugar and some chocolate biscuits. He improved a bit almost immediately, but was still very disorientated. I got someone else to ring his home and we sat him in the station until his wife fetched him. He wrote to me later and said he thought the cause was working late and only having a light lunch that day. 🙿

WHAT TO DO:

1 Recognise the symptoms: fainting, odourless breath, dizziness, difficulty with eyesight, tremors, possibly aggressive or bizarre behaviour.

2 Look for a diabetic bracelet, tag or card.

3 Offer sugar immediately: sugar lumps, biscuits, fruit juice, cake, fizzy drink (with sugar, not a 'diet' drink with saccharine).

4 If the casualty becomes unconscious before or in spite of your help, open his airway, put him in the Recovery Position (see **p 22**) and send for an ambulance.

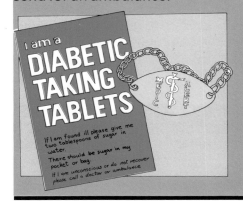

STROKE:

> *I was watching television and got up to change channels – that was all – when I had my stroke. It was all very frightening, but I stayed more or less conscious throughout. What made such a difference was how calm and unpanicked my wife and daughters were. They sent for an ambulance within seconds, or so it seemed, held my hand and murmured cheerful soothing things to me. I knew there was nothing else they could do, but it made all the difference in the world that there was absolutely no chaos. I'm sure it's one of the reasons I made such a good recovery.*

The signs of a stroke may include inability to move limbs on one side of the body, difficulty in speech, breathing and swallowing, and unequal pupil size. In a severe stroke the casualty may become unconscious.

WHAT TO DO:

1 If the victim is conscious, reassure him, and make him comfortable by propping up his head and shoulders. Turn his head slightly to one side so that any saliva dribbling from the mouth will drain away.

2 Send for an ambulance.

3   While you are waiting for the ambulance, treat the casualty for shock (see **p 64**) by keeping him warm and raising his legs above chest level.

4   If he is unconscious, open the airway and turn him into the Recovery Position (see **p 22**).

EPILEPTIC FITS:

Claire Hann was only five when she acted promptly enough to save her mother Debra from possible suffocation after an epileptic fit at home. She calmed her two little sisters down and between them they managed to half-turn Debra into the Recovery Position. Claire also found and used correctly the special plastic airway that she had seen ambulancemen use when they had been called previously to help her mother. Only then did she dial 999 and ring both sets of grandparents. Such collected and sensible behaviour is rare in adults, let alone in such a young child, and Claire certainly deserved the 'Children of Courage' award she received.

An epileptic fit – a very common emergency involving electrical disturbances in the brain – is much less mysterious and frightening than at first it seems. However, an epileptic is potentially at risk if unconsciousness lasts for more than a few minutes. Epileptics also suffer as a result of the fear of bystanders:

> **"** *I came across a woman lying on the ground outside a small rank of shops in Ealing. She was jerking and twitching and it was obvious to me that she was having an epileptic fit. Because she looked scruffy, people were walking right round her, carefully wheeling their shopping baskets the while, assuming she was drunk. One of the shopkeepers came rushing out and started trying to force her mouth open. Fortunately the woman's boyfriend stopped him. She came round after about five minutes.* **"**

The signs of a fit are:

- Unconsciousness.
- Stiffening of the arms, legs and neck, followed by violent shaking and twitching.
- Clenching of the teeth and noisy or difficult breathing.
- The sufferer may wet or soil himself.
- The sufferer may bite his tongue or froth at the mouth.
- The muscles then relax, though usually he will remain unconscious for a few more minutes.

WHAT TO DO:

1 There may be some warning of what is to happen: the sufferer may shout or cry, or stagger – if so, try to break his fall by catching him.

2 Don't let people crowd around.

3 Look for an identity tag, bracelet or card which may tell you how long his fits usually last.

4 Protect him as far as you can from hurting himself during the jerking stage of the fit, but don't try to restrain him: just move anything away that might hurt him.

5 Don't try to put anything into his mouth – this can be dangerous.

6 When the jerking stops, turn him into the Recovery Position (see **p 22**) as he will probably still be unconscious.

7 When he comes round, leave him where he is for a few minutes, reassure him, then make sure that he rests quietly for at least an hour afterwards.

8   In most cases there is no need to call an
    ambulance. Call an ambulance only if:

- There are several fits one after the other
  without the victim regaining consciousness.
- The victim has suffered a bad injury in the
  fall or during the convulsions.

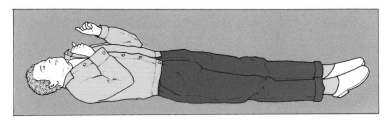

**An epileptic in the jerking stage of a fit may well
adopt this position. Don't try to restrain him: just
move away anything that might hurt him.**

HYPOTHERMIA:

This is a condition where body temperature drops dangerously low. If left untreated, it results in unconsciousness and then death. Three groups of people are the most vulnerable: babies sleeping in cold bedrooms, the elderly who may be neglecting themselves, and sportsmen and sportswomen whose sport (especially mountaineering, pot-holing or swimming) may expose them to unusually cold conditions for a long time.

Someone suffering from hypothermia will feel unnaturally cold if you touch her and she may shiver uncontrollably. Gradually the intense shivering slows down and so do her breathing and pulse. Eventually unconsciousness takes over. Extreme hypothermia is usually fatal, but the outlook is good in less severe cases as long as you give help promptly.

Babies suffering from hypothermia have misleadingly pink faces, hands and feet, but their skin feels intensely cold and they are drowsy and limp. Treat them in the same way as adults.

WHAT TO DO:

Your main aim is to warm the victim up quickly, but this must be done in the right way:

1 Find a warm blanket, rug, eiderdown or duvet and wrap her in it. Cover her head (a quarter of our body heat is lost through the head), but leave her face clear. Alternatively, put her in a warm, hand-hot bath, as long as she is completely conscious and only at the

shivering stage. Do not leave her alone; stay with her, supporting her shoulders.

2 If possible, warm the room up quickly – for example, with a fan heater – or move her to an already warmer room.

3 Give a conscious casualty something hot to drink.

4 If she is unconscious, put her in the Recovery Position (see **p 22**). Keep checking her breathing and pulse, and be prepared to resuscitate.

5 If you have to attempt resuscitation, check even more carefully than usual for a pulse. The reason is that her pulse may be slow and irregular. Chest compression can be particularly dangerous to a hypothermia casualty whose heart is still beating.

6 Don't stop the attempt to resuscitate, however hopeless it seems. With hypothermia all the body processes slow right down: many apparently dead patients have recovered when they have been warmed up.

It is important not to draw blood away from the vital organs to the skin, so:

DON'T encourage exercise.

DON'T rub the victim's legs or arms.

You can use a hot water bottle as long as it is well wrapped and put on the casualty's trunk, not her arms or legs.

LEARNING MORE:

In this book we have tried to describe all the basic elements of emergency life-saving. Read it through frequently and keep it in a place where you can refer to it quickly. For further reading, we recommend the First Aid Manual (Dorling Kindersley), published jointly by the three voluntary aid societies – the St John Ambulance, the Red Cross and St Andrew's Ambulance Association. This comprehensive, reasonably priced and well-illustrated guide to every kind of first aid includes advice on dealing with minor but unpleasant emergencies (for instance, fainting, small burns) as well as some major but uncommon ones (for instance, bullet wounds and snake bites) which we have excluded from this book.

However, there is a limit to what can be learnt from books alone. To feel really prepared to cope, you should consider going to a class. The advantages are:

1 Learning by doing is always the best way of remembering. As the old Chinese proverb says:

I hear and I forget
I see and I remember
I do and I understand

The truth of this proverb has been proved many times in educational experiments. Once you have actually carried out mouth-to-mouth resuscitation in the correct way, it is much easier to remember the technique than if you have merely read about it in a book. Moreover, at a class you will have access to a manikin (dummy) specially designed for teaching. This will give you the chance to practise chest compression, a technique which it is positively dangerous to practise on a living person whose heart is

118

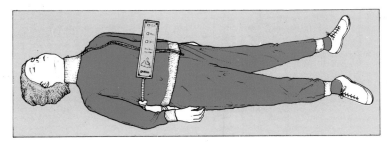

A training manikin of the type used in emergency aid classes.

beating normally. You will also be able to practise mouth-to-mouth breathing on the manikin; this is not so much dangerous as unpleasant and, perhaps, embarrassing to try on fellow class members. Practising on a manikin takes away the embarrassment.

2 Mistakes can be corrected. There are some aspects of emergency first aid where it is hard to know whether your actions are correct or not. For example, are you actually pressing the right place on the chest? Have you extended the neck too far or not far enough in trying to open the airway? How hard do you really pull with the Heimlich manoeuvre? In a class, because the tutor is there to help you, any mistakes can be very easily put right.

3 Learning resuscitation as a sequence. One of the best reasons for going to a class is that you will learn a complete procedure and practise it as a sequence. Most people find this helpful and it has proved its value in a real emergency time and time again. Here are the experiences of two rescuers who had attended classes:

> **"**
>
> *I didn't stop to think. I just swung straight into it – Assess the casualty. Is he conscious? Open his airway . . . is he breathing? Give mouth-to-mouth, and so on. Afterwards I rang my tutor to thank him for making us all go through the whole thing so many times – it obviously sank in.*
>
> **"**

❝

It came flooding back to me: 'A for Airway, B for Breathing, C for Circulation' – I just did it. I could hear our teacher's voice droning on: 'Shake and shout. Unconscious? You must open the airway . . .' I don't think I would have remembered it as well as I did without having practised it in a class. **❞**

4   Asking questions. Many people enrol for a class because they have already been involved in a taxing emergency. Going to a class will give you the opportunity to discuss such an experience with other people, and also to have an expert on hand to answer your questions. This has proved a good way for some students to come to terms with an experience which may have left them feeling confused or guilty. One person who had attended classes recalled:

❝

I was able to ask the woman taking the class about the circumstances in which my father died. She pointed out something which was obvious, really: that there was no purpose in reproaching myself for what I hadn't known then. Several of the other people there had similar tales to tell and I felt a lot happier about it all, not least because I knew I would be so much better prepared to deal with a similar incident in the future. **❞**

A class is also a good place to ask about special circumstances which may be worrying you. What about asthmatics? What about someone who has arthritis in her neck – can her airway be opened? Does a diagnosis of 'angina' mean that a heart attack is inevitable?

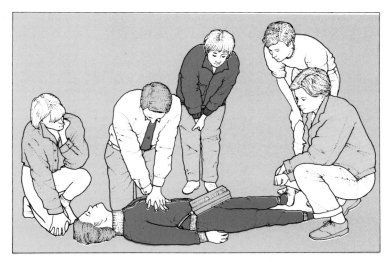

Chest compressions being demonstrated on a manikin.

How to find a class

Learning first aid has gone through a considerable revolution in the last ten years. Before that, the only certain way of getting face-to-face teaching was to enrol on a Red Cross, St John Ambulance or St Andrew's Ambulance Association course, normally meeting one evening a week over several weeks. Since 1978, thanks to pioneering work in Brighton (which in its turn was inspired by pioneering work in America), the simple single-session two-hour class has established its place as an attractive alternative. It appeals to people who just want to learn the basics of resuscitation, and also to those who, whatever their good intentions, can never find the time to undertake the full first aid course.

Most of the original two-hour courses were run by hospitals, where an energetic consultant from the Accident and Emergency, Anaesthetics or Cardiology Department set up his own 'community education' scheme. Now, thanks to the 'Save A Life' campaign, it should be possible to find a two-hour class in most areas, though some are much better served than others. 'Save A Life' classes may be run by the local education authority as part of their normal adult education service, by a local hospital or health education service, by one of the voluntary first aid societies, by the Royal Life Saving Society, or by companies for their employees.

To find a two-hour 'Save A Life' class you could try any of these routes:

● Telephone your local education authority (the number is in your local directory) and ask the adult education office whether they are running classes.

● Telephone your local branch of the Red Cross, St John Ambulance or St Andrew's Ambulance Association. The Red Cross is entered in the phone book under 'British Red Cross Society'.

● In some areas schemes are run from a local hospital. Usually these local campaigns have their own special names (for instance, in Wakefield, 'The Wakefield Life Support Scheme'; in Brighton, 'Heartguard'). They publicise their activities very thoroughly and run regular 'open' sessions where you can simply book in by telephone.

● Some Royal Life Saving Society branches run two-hour resuscitation courses.

● Your employer may be willing to sponsor a scheme. Responsible employers are highly aware of the need to expand the number of people who know what to do in a medical emergency. Large companies employ safety experts who are responsible for organising first aid training. They may be willing to organize courses themselves if approached. Alternatively, if you have an active 'Save A Life' campaign locally, its co-ordinator may be willing to visit your company and run a course on site.

● Write to the 'Save A Life' campaign at the Royal Society of Medicine, 1 Wimpole Street, London W1, for details of classes in your area. Please enclose a stamped self-addressed envelope.

Taking it further

Doing a two-hour course will help you learn the basics of resuscitation. If you want to know more about the wider subject of first aid, there are longer first aid courses run by all the voluntary aid societies. There are two main types of course:

● A weekly class meeting for two or three hours a week over a period of weeks, with an optional exam at the end of it. This is one of the ways in which, for instance, the St John Ambulance prepares its volunteers for their work as those familiar figures in black and white uniform at public events.

● An intensive three- or four-day course normally run for employees who want to become first aiders at their place of work. The exam at the end of the course must be taken to qualify as a first aider who meets the Health and Safety Executive's stringent requirements. If you wish to continue as a first aider, the exam must be re-taken after a brief refresher course every three years.

For details of courses, write (enclosing a stamped, self-addressed envelope) to the national headquarters of any of the voluntary aid societies:

British Red Cross Society
9 Grosvenor Crescent
London
SW1 7EJ
Telephone: 01–235 5454

St Andrew's Ambulance Association
St Andrew's House
Milton Street
Glasgow
G4 0HR
Telephone: 041–332 4031

St John Ambulance
1 Grosvenor Crescent
London
SW1X 7EF
Telephone: 01–235 5231

For more information on emergency aid classes, write, enclosing an s.a.e., to:

Royal Life Saving Society UK
Mountbatten House
Studley
Warwickshire
B80 7NN

'Save A Life' Campaign
Royal Society of Medicine
1 Wimpole Street
London W1

Resuscitation Council (UK)
c/o Dept of Anaesthetics
Royal Postgraduate Medical School
Ducane Road
London W12

INDEX: